Pediatric Craniofacial Surgery: State of the Craft

Editor

EDWARD P. BUCHANAN

CLINICS IN PLASTIC SURGERY

www.plasticsurgery.theclinics.com

April 2019 • Volume 46 • Number 2

ELSEVIER

1600 John F. Kennedy Boulevard ● Suite 1800 ● Philadelphia, Pennsylvania, 19103-2899

http://www.theclinics.com

CLINICS IN PLASTIC SURGERY Volume 46, Number 2
April 2019 ISSN 0094-1298, ISBN-13: 978-0-323-65570-5

Editor: Jessica McCool
Developmental Editor: Meredith Madeira

Clinics in Plastic Surgery (ISSN 0094-1298) is published quarterly by Elsevier Inc., 360 Park Avenue South, New York, NY 10010-1710. Months of issue are January, April, July, and October. Business and Editorial Offices: 1600 John F. Kennedy Blvd., Suite 1800, Philadelphia, PA 19103-2899. Periodicals postage paid at New York, NY and additional mailing offices. Subscription prices are $543.00 per year for US individuals, $940.00 per year for US institutions, $100.00 per year for US students and residents, $607.00 per year for Canadian individuals, $1119.00 per year for Canadian institutions, $649.00 per year for international individuals, $1119.00 per year for international institutions, and $305.00 per year for Canadian and international students/residents. To receive student/resident rate, orders must be accompanied by name of affiliated institution, date of term, and the *signature* of program/residency coordinator on institution letterhead. Orders will be billed at individual rate until proof of status is received. Foreign air speed delivery is included in all *Clinics* subscription prices. All prices are subject to change without notice. **POSTMASTER:** Send address changes to *Clinics in Plastic Surgery*, Elsevier Health Sciences Division, Subscription Customer Service, 3251 Riverport Lane, Maryland Heights, MO 63043. **Customer Service: 1-800-654-2452 (US and Canada). From outside of the United States and Canada, call 314-447-8871. Fax: 314-447-8029. E-mail: JournalsCustomerService-usa@elsevier.com (for print support); JournalsOnlineSupport-usa@ elsevier.com (for online support).**

Reprints. For copies of 100 or more of articles in this publication, please contact the Commercial Reprints Department, Elsevier Inc., 360 Park Avenue South, New York, New York 10010-1710. Tel.: +1-212-633-3874; Fax: +1-212-633-3820; E-mail: reprints@elsevier.com.

Clinics in Plastic Surgery is covered in *Current Contents, EMBASE/Excerpta Medica, Science Citation Index, MEDLINE/ PubMed (Index Medicus), ASCA, and ISI/BIOMED.*

Contributors

EDITOR

EDWARD P. BUCHANAN, MD, FACS
Chief, Division of Plastic Surgery, Director of
Cleft Care, Program Director of Craniofacial
Fellowship, Texas Children's Hospital,
Associate Professor, Division of Plastic
Surgery, Michael E. DeBakey Department of
Surgery, Baylor College of Medicine, Houston,
Texas, USA

AUTHORS

ALBARAA ALJERIAN, MBBS
Resident, Division of Plastic and
Reconstructive Surgery, McGill University
Health Center, Montreal, Quebec,
Canada

TOM W. ANDREW, MBChB, MSc
Hagey Laboratory for Pediatric Regenerative
Medicine, Division of Plastic Surgery,
Department of Surgery, Stanford University,
School of Medicine, Stanford, California,
USA

CRAIG BIRGFELD, MD, FACS
Associate Professor, Pediatric Plastic
and Craniofacial Surgery, Seattle
Children's Hospital, Seattle, Washington,
USA

EDWARD P. BUCHANAN, MD, FACS
Chief, Division of Plastic Surgery, Director of
Cleft Care, Program Director of Craniofacial
Fellowship, Texas Children's Hospital,
Associate Professor, Division of Plastic
Surgery, Michael E. DeBakey Department of
Surgery, Baylor College of Medicine, Houston,
Texas, USA

MICHAEL R. BYKOWSKI, MD, MS
Integrated Plastic Surgery Resident,
Department of Plastic Surgery, University of
Pittsburgh Medical Center, Pittsburgh,
Pennsylvania, USA

DANIEL C. CHELIUS Jr, MD
Assistant Professor, Pediatric Otolaryngology–
Head and Neck Surgery, Baylor College of
Medicine, Houston, Texas, USA

ROBERT C. DAUSER, MD
Associate Professor, Department of
Neurosurgery, Baylor College of Medicine,
Houston, Texas, USA

ROBERT F. DEMPSEY, MD
Assistant Professor, Division of Plastic
Surgery, Michael E. DeBakey Department of
Surgery, Baylor College of Medicine, Houston,
Texas, USA

AMY L. DIMACHKIEH, MD
Assistant Professor, Pediatric Otolaryngology–
Head and Neck Surgery, Baylor College of
Medicine, Houston, Texas, USA

ELAINE DONG, BA
Division of Plastic Surgery, Baylor College of
Medicine, Houston, Texas, USA

**MIRKO S. GILARDINO, MD, MSc, FRCSC,
FACS**
Director, H.B. Williams Craniofacial and Cleft
Surgery Unit, Montreal Children's Hospital,
Associate Professor of Surgery, Division of
Plastic and Reconstructive Surgery, McGill
University Health Center, Montreal, Quebec,
Canada

JESSE A. GOLDSTEIN, MD, FACS, FAAP
Assistant Professor, Department of Plastic
Surgery, Children's Hospital of Pittsburgh of
University of Pittsburgh Medical Center,
Pittsburgh, Pennsylvania, USA

CARRIE HEIKE, MD, MS
Craniofacial Pediatrics, Seattle Children's
Hospital, Seattle, Washington, USA

LARRY H. HOLLIER Jr, MD
Professor, Division of Plastic Surgery,
Michael E. DeBakey Department of Surgery,
Baylor College of Medicine, Houston, Texas,
USA

IAN C. HOPPE, MD
Fellow, Division of Plastic Surgery, University of
Pennsylvania, Philadelphia, Pennsylvania, USA

SUN T. HSIEH, MS, MD
Chief Resident, Department of Plastic Surgery,
Rhode Island Hospital, The Warren Alpert
Medical School of Brown University,
Providence, Rhode Island, USA

MICHAEL E. KUPFERMAN, MD
Professor, Department of Head and Neck
Surgery, Division of Surgery, The University of
Texas MD Anderson Cancer Center, Houston,
Texas, USA

SANDI K. LAM, MD
Associate Professor, Department of
Neurosurgery, Baylor College of Medicine,
Houston, Texas, USA

H. PETER LORENZ, MD
Professor of Plastic Surgery, Service Chief,
Plastic Surgery, Lucile Packard Children's
Hospital, Director, Craniofacial Surgery
Fellowship, Division of Plastic Surgery,
Department of Surgery, Stanford University
School of Medicine, Stanford, California, USA

JOSEPH E. LOSEE, MD, FACS, FAAP
Dr. Ross H. Musgrave Endowed Chair in
Pediatric Plastic Surgery, Associate Dean for
Faculty Affairs, University of Pittsburgh School
of Medicine, Professor and Executive Vice
Chair, Department of Plastic Surgery, Division
Chief, Pediatric Plastic Surgery, Children's
Hospital of Pittsburgh of University of
Pittsburgh Medical Center, Pittsburgh,
Pennsylvania, USA

MARCO MARICEVICH, MD
Assistant Professor, Division of Plastic
Surgery, Michael E. DeBakey Department of
Surgery, Baylor College of Medicine, Houston,
Texas, USA

RENATA S. MARICEVICH, MD
Assistant Professor, Division of Plastic
Surgery, Michael E. DeBakey Department of
Surgery, Baylor College of Medicine, Houston,
Texas, USA

LAURA A. MONSON, MD
Assistant Professor, Division of Plastic
Surgery, Michael E. DeBakey Department of
Surgery, Baylor College of Medicine, Houston,
Texas, USA

ROSHAN MORBIA, MD
Craniofacial Surgery Fellow, Division of Plastic
Surgery, Department of Surgery, Stanford
University, School of Medicine, Stanford,
California, USA

SHOLA OLARUNNIPA, MD
Assistant Professor, Division of Plastic
Surgery, Michael E. DeBakey Department of
Surgery, Baylor College of Medicine, Houston,
Texas, USA

WILLIAM C. PEDERSON, MD
Associate Professor, Division of Plastic
Surgery, Michael E. DeBakey Department of
Surgery, Baylor College of Medicine, Houston,
Texas, USA

JOHN PHILLIPS, BSc, MA, MD, FRCSC
Associate Professor, Division of Plastic and
Reconstructive Surgery, University of Toronto,
Hospital for Sick Children, Toronto, Ontario,
Canada

JOHN REINISCH, MD, FACS
Professor of Surgery, Keck School of Medicine
of USC, University of Southern California,
Cedars-Sinai Medical Center, Los Angeles,
California, USA

ANDREE-ANNE ROY, MD, MSc, FRCSC
Clinical Fellow, Department of Plastic
and Reconstructive Surgery, Hospital
for Sick Children, Toronto, Ontario,
Canada

MICHAEL ALEXANDER RTSHILADZE, BSc (Med), MBBS, MS, FRACS
Plastic Surgeon, Craniofacial Unit, Department of Plastic and Reconstructive Surgery, Sydney Children's Hospital, Randwick, Sydney, New South Wales, Australia

RAJENDRA SAWH-MARTINEZ, MD, MHS
Craniofacial Fellow, Section of Plastic and Reconstructive Surgery, Department of Surgery, Yale University, New Haven, Connecticut, USA

KELLY P. SCHULTZ, BA
Division of Plastic Surgery, Baylor College of Medicine, Houston, Texas, USA

SAMEER SHAKIR, MD
Resident, Division of Plastic Surgery, University of Pennsylvania, Philadelphia, Pennsylvania, USA

DEREK M. STEINBACHER, DMD, MD, FACS
Associate Professor, Section of Plastic and Reconstructive Surgery, Director of Craniofacial Surgery, Chief of Dentistry, Chief of Oral and Maxillofacial Surgery, Department of Surgery, Yale New Haven Hospital, Yale University, New Haven, Connecticut, USA

KYLE STEVENS, BSc, DDS, MSc, FRCDC
Orthodontist, Orthodontics, Department of Dentistry, Hospital for Sick Children, Toronto, Ontario, Canada

YOUSSEF TAHIRI, MD, MSc, FRCSC, FAAP, FACS
Associate Professor of Surgery, Craniofacial and Pediatric Plastic Surgery, Cedars-Sinai Medical Center, Los Angeles, California, USA

JESSE A. TAYLOR, MD
Peter Randall Endowed Chair and Chief, Division of Plastic Surgery, The Children's Hospital of Philadelphia, Philadelphia, Pennsylvania, USA

TUAN A. TRUONG, MD
Assistant Professor, Division of Plastic Surgery, Michael E. DeBakey Department of Surgery, Baylor College of Medicine, Houston, Texas, USA

HOWARD L. WEINER, MD
Professor, Division of Pediatric Neurosurgery, Michael E. DeBakey Department of Surgery, Baylor College of Medicine, Houston, Texas, USA

ALBERT S. WOO, MD, FACS
Division Chief, Pediatric Plastic Surgery, Director, Craniofacial Program, Associate Professor of Surgery, Pediatrics and Neurosurgery, Rhode Island Hospital, The Warren Alpert Medical School of Brown University, Providence, Rhode Island, USA

Contents

Nonsyndromic craniosynostosis is significantly more common than syndromic craniosynostosis, affecting the sagittal, coronal, metopic, and lambdoid sutures in decreasing order of frequency. Nonsyndromic craniosynostosis is most frequently associated with only 1 fused suture, creating a predictable head shape. Repair of craniosynostosis is recommended to avoid potential neurodevelopmental delay. Early intervention at 3 to 4 months of age allows minimally invasive approaches, but requires postoperative molding helmet therapy and good family compliance. Open techniques are deferred until the child is older to better tolerate the associated surgical stress. Cranial vault remodeling is generally well-tolerated with a low rate of complications.

Management strategies for syndromic craniosynostosis patients require multidisciplinary subspecialty teams to provide optimal care for complex reconstructive approaches. The most common craniosynostosis syndromes include Apert (FGFR2), Crouzon (FGFR2), Muenke (FGFR3), Pfeiffer (FGFR1 and FGFR2), and Saethre-Chotzen (TWIST). Bicoronal craniosynostosis (turribrachycephaly) is most commonly associated with syndromic craniosynostosis. Disease presentation varies from mild sutural involvement to severe pansynostoses, with a spectrum of extracraniofacial dysmorphic manifestations. Understanding the multifaceted syndromic presentations while appreciating the panoply of variable presentations is central to delivering necessary individualized care. Cranial vault remodeling aims to relieve restriction of cranial development and elevated intracranial pressure and restore normal morphology.

Cleft orthognathic surgery is an important component of a comprehensive cleft care plan. Applying combined orthodontic and orthognathic treatment principles to a cohort of patients with cleft lip and palate raises many challenges not encountered in conventional orthognathic care. Cleft patients share a commonality in their midfacial anatomy that is characterized by a 3-dimensionally deficient maxilla. The residual sequelae of multiple previous surgeries along with dental differences and unhealed fistulae are considerations when embarking on treatment. This article describes many of these challenges and highlights approaches that are used to address the specific needs of this special group of patients.

and psychological trauma. Excellent outcomes with minimal morbidity can be obtained using this technique. This type of microtia reconstruction provides a more holistic approach because it is done at a younger age, in a single stage, as an outpatient and could address the functional hearing issues earlier.

Parry-Romberg syndrome, or progressive hemifacial atrophy, is a rare disorder of unknown etiology. Patients present with unilateral atrophy of skin that may progress to involve underlying fat, muscle, and osseocartilaginous structures. Neurologic complications are common. After self-limited disease stabilization, various reconstructive options may be used to restore patients' facial symmetry. Serial autologous fat grafting has shown favorable results in reconstruction of mild or moderate soft tissue deficiency, but free tissue transfer remains the treatment of choice for severe disease.

Pediatric facial fracture management is often complex and demanding. The structure and topography of the pediatric craniofacial skeleton are profoundly different from the mature skull. Consequently, the pediatric facial skeleton responds differently to traumatic force. Although the incidence of pediatric facial trauma is higher than in the adult population, the incidence of facial fracture is significantly lower. The management in younger patients is often more conservative because of potential growth impairment. As the facial skeleton matures, more conventional surgical approaches become appropriate. This review provides an understanding of the unique elements of facial fracture management in the pediatric population.

 Video content accompanies this article at http://www.plasticsurgery.theclinics.com.

Pierre Robin sequence consists of clinical triad of micrognathia, glossoptosis, and airway compromise with variable inclusion of cleft palate. Evaluation of airway obstruction includes physical examination, polysomnography for obstruction events, and a combination of nasoendoscopy and bronchoscopy to search for synchronous obstructive lesions. A multidisciplinary approach is required given the high rate of syndromic disease. Management of airway obstruction and feeding starts with nonsurgical maneuvers, such as prone and lateral positioning, nasopharyngeal stenting, and continuous positive airway pressure. Surgical management includes mandibular distraction and tongue-lip adhesion. Subglottic obstruction and central sleep apnea may best be treated with tracheostomy.

Reconstruction of defects of the head and face in the pediatric population requires special consideration for future growth, and at times temporization in anticipation for skeletal maturity followed by subsequent reoperation at an appropriate age. Additional challenges include more limited donor sites, smaller anastomoses, and unpredictable postoperative compliance compared with their adult counterparts. Nonetheless, successful composite bony and soft tissue, and isolated soft tissue defects in children are safely reconstructed using existing local tissue and microsurgical techniques.

CLINICS IN PLASTIC SURGERY

ISSUE OF RELATED INTEREST

Facial Plastic Surgery Clinics of North America,
Volume 26, Issue 1 (February 2018)
Cosmetic and Reconstructive Surgery of Congenital Ear Deformities
Scott Stephan, *Editor*

THE CLINICS ARE AVAILABLE ONLINE!
Access your subscription at:
www.theclinics.com

Preface

Pediatric Craniofacial Surgery: State of the Craft

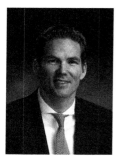

Edward P. Buchanan, MD, FACS
Editor

As a specialized discipline within the field of medicine, pediatric craniofacial surgery is in its infancy. Dr Paul Tessier began his monumental work and created this practice just over 60 years ago. Since that time, it has become widely adapted and practiced all over the world. Whereas his original techniques have been modified and advanced, the spirit of his initial goals is very much alive. This issue of *Clinics in Plastic Surgery* reviews the current state of the practice from a diverse population of authors who are experts in their respective fields. This issue not only is intended as an overview, but also provides a closer look into the specifics of some of the most complex types of surgical interventions currently offered. What becomes apparent upon reviewing each of these articles is the amount of advancement we have achieved as a specialty in the last 60 years. Despite these successes, there remains a tremendous amount of work to do to provide an even greater level of care for our patients to improve the quality and outcomes of our work. Understanding the limits of our profession and finding the edge of our knowledge will help our current and future leaders redefine these boundaries for the benefit of our patients and our profession.

Edward P. Buchanan, MD, FACS
Division of Plastic Surgery
Texas Children's Hospital
Baylor College of Medicine
6701 Fannin Street
Suite 610.00
Houston, TX 77030, USA

E-mail address:
ebuchana@bcm.edu

Clin Plastic Surg 46 (2019) xiii
https://doi.org/10.1016/j.cps.2018.12.002
0094-1298/19/© 2018 Published by Elsevier Inc.

Nonsyndromic Craniosynostosis

Robert F. Dempsey, MD[a], Laura A. Monson, MD[a], Renata S. Maricevich, MD[a],
Tuan A. Truong, MD[a], Shola Olarunnipa, MD[a], Sandi K. Lam, MD[b], Robert C. Dauser, MD[b],
Larry H. Hollier Jr, MD[a], Edward P. Buchanan, MD[a],*

KEYWORDS

- Nonsyndromic craniosynostosis • Craniosynostosis • Cranial suture • Cranial vault remodeling
- Pediatric craniofacial surgery

KEY POINTS

- Nonsyndromic craniosynostosis is significantly more common than syndromic craniosynostosis, affecting the sagittal, coronal, metopic, and lambdoid sutures in decreasing order of frequency.
- A majority of nonsyndromic craniosynostosis case involve only 1 suture.
- Single suture craniosynostosis produces a predictable head shape, allowing for diagnosis from physical examination findings.
- Repair of craniosynostosis is generally recommended to avoid potential neurodevelopmental delay.
- Early intervention of craniosynostosis at 3 to 4 months of age may be done through minimally invasive methods, but requires a course of postoperative molding helmet therapy and subsequent good family compliance.

INTRODUCTION

Abnormal head shape is a common reason for referral to the pediatric or craniofacial plastic surgeon. Deformational plagiocephaly continues to be the most common reason for abnormal pediatric head shape, which has been estimated to occur at a frequency as high as 46.6% since the introduction of the American Academy of Pediatrics "Back to Sleep" campaign in 1992.[1] Efforts to increase education among our pediatrician colleagues has been largely successful in accurate diagnosis without specialist referral. However, when the diagnosis remains in question or craniosynostosis is suspected by the pediatrician, the child should be promptly referred to a craniofacial team for assessment.

Timely diagnosis of craniosynostosis, defined as premature fusion of the cranial sutures, is important to allow interventions to prevent the development of intracranial hypertension, which can affect neurodevelopment. Currently, the diagnosis of craniosynostosis is subdivided between involvement of a single versus multiple sutures and/or syndromic versus nonsyndromic craniosynostosis. Syndromic craniosynostosis is associated with other anomalies of the face, trunk, or limbs and generally involves multiple cranial sutures. Discussion of syndromic craniosynostosis is beyond the scope of this article.

In contrast, nonsyndromic craniosynostosis usually involves only one of the following sutures listed in decreasing order of frequency: sagittal, coronal, metopic, and lambdoid. Owing to this generalization, single suture and nonsyndromic craniosynostosis designations are commonly used interchangeably. However, this is technically inaccurate, and although rare, nonsyndromic multiple

Disclosure Statement: The authors have nothing to disclose.
[a] Division of Plastic Surgery, Michael E. DeBakey Department of Surgery, Baylor College of Medicine, 6701 Fannin Street, CC 610.00, Houston, TX 77030, USA; [b] Department of Neurosurgery, Baylor College of Medicine, 6701 Fannin Street, CC 1230.01, Houston, TX 77030, USA
* Corresponding author.
E-mail address: ebuchana@bcm.edu

Clin Plastic Surg 46 (2019) 123–139
https://doi.org/10.1016/j.cps.2018.11.001
0094-1298/19/© 2018 Elsevier Inc. All rights reserved.

suture craniosynostoses do exist and categorized as complex nonsyndromic craniosynostosis.

Overall, craniosynostosis occurs in 1 in 2500 births. In a recent study, 84% of patients presented with isolated craniosynostosis, 7% with additional clinical symptoms and 9% with suspected syndromic craniosynostosis. This correlates with a nonsyndromic craniosynostosis incidence of 0.4 to 1.0 in 1000 births.[2] Interestingly, there is a different gender predisposition among sagittal and unicoronal synostosis patients, with sagittal synostosis occurring more commonly in males at a rate of 4:1 and unicoronal synostosis occurring more commonly in females at a rate of 3:2.[2]

The underlying genetic origin of pathologic premature suture fusion continues to be a point of focused research. Mutations in both the FGF-2 and TGF-β genes have been implicated in craniosynostosis of murine models. These genes are often specifically tested for when syndromic craniosynostosis is suspected, but have also been associated with nonsyndromic disease.[3,4] As our understanding of how these genes regulate the interaction between the cranial bones, dura, and timing of suture fusion improves, we may one day design targeted therapies to avoid craniosynostosis.

When evaluating the craniosynostosis patient, even the nonsyndromic patient, a multidisciplinary craniofacial team approach is best. Most craniofacial teams are championed by a team coordinator, who functions as the liaison between the patient and the treating team. This individual gives the family a common point of contact to coordinate all care needs. Additional team members consist of craniofacial and neurosurgeons, ophthalmologists, otolaryngologists, and geneticists among others as discussed elsewhere in this article (**Box 1**).[5]

Although many families of craniosynostosis children present to the craniofacial surgeon desiring restoration of normal head shape for primarily aesthetic reasons, the primary indication for intervention is to prevent the sequela of intracranial hypertension (defined as >15 mm Hg). Intracranial hypertension can result in neurodevelopmental delay, although its exact incidence is not well-understood. The most recent studies indicate a 15% incidence of intracranial hypertension.[6] However, resultant neurodevelopmental delay is more difficult to determine and likely multifactorial, including the presence of hydrocephalus, structural changes of the brain, prematurity, and family history. Some studies have indicated evidence of neurodevelopmental delay in single suture craniosynostosis patients to be as high as 37%.[7]

> **Box 1**
> **List of craniofacial team members**
>
> *Multidisciplinary Craniofacial Team Members*
> Audiologists
> Dentists/Orthodontists
> Otolaryngologists
> Ophthalmologists
> Geneticists and Genetic Counselors
> Neurosurgeons
> Nurse Practitioners
> Nurses
> Nutritionists
> Occupational/Physical Therapists
> Oral and Maxillofacial Surgeons
> Pediatricians
> Plastic and Reconstructive Surgeons
> Psychologists
> Researchers
> Respiratory Therapists
> Social Workers
> Speech and Language Pathologists
> Support Staff

To further confound this issue, even if the true incidence of craniosynostosis-associated neurodevelopmental delay were determined, we are currently unable to reliably predict which children will be affected. Thus, the current paradigm recommends surgical correction of the condition in all children. For families particularly reluctant to pursue initial surgery, close follow-up with serial dilated eye examinations to detect the presence of papilledema, and associated intracranial hypertension may be offered. If detected, surgical intervention is strongly indicated.

The timing of surgical intervention is another topic of much debate. For nonsyndromic children, surgery is usually deferred until at least 3 months of age, which is thought to allow the child to better compensate to physiologic stress of bleeding. Although the volume of blood lost during surgery is usually not excessive, it comprises a proportionally greater percentage of the baby's developing total blood pool than older patients. In general, surgery is defined as early or late, which is defined as greater than 1 year of life.

Early intervention within the first 3 to 4 months of life is required for endoscopic repair to take advantage of the rapidly growing brain during helmet therapy, which is discussed elsewhere in this article. In addition to the benefit of brain growth on head shape, advocates of early intervention for open repair also point to the benefit of preventing further progression of secondary craniofacial changes as well as more easily molded bone stock. Additionally, children who undergo early intervention are more likely to spontaneously reossify any residual calvarial defects. Proponents of late intervention point to the increased rate of revision required in the early intervention children.

In practice, most surgeons intervene in at between 3 and 12 months of age, and this decision is affected by technique and surgeon bias. Herein we present the practice adopted by the senior author and our institution.

PREOPERATIVE EVALUATION

Upon initial evaluation, children undergo a routine history and physical examination. Physical examination by the experienced clinician is sufficient to differentiate between positional and deformational plagiocephaly. If positional plagiocephaly is diagnosed, reassurance is provided to the family and appropriate referrals to occupational therapy for treatment of underlying torticollis or molding helmet therapy are made as indicated.

Beyond differentiating between positional and deformational plagiocephaly, the type of craniosynostosis present is easily made due to the characteristic head shape premature single suture fusion produces. This finding is based on work by Virchow, who in 1851 made the landmark observation that premature suture fusion results in a predictable compensatory perpendicular growth in the unaffected skull (**Fig. 1**). These various calvarial deformations are discussed in further detail elsewhere in the article.[8]

If craniosynostosis is suspected, referral to neuroophthalmology is made for visual assessment, including a dilated eye examination, because abnormalities are commonly associated.[9] If not already obtained, imaging via noncontrasted craniofacial computed tomography with 3-dimensional reconstruction is obtained. Originally, routine imaging was controversial owing to concerns of unnecessary radiation exposure to the child. However, current rapid low-dose craniofacial computed tomgoraphy protocols have largely eliminated this concern with reduction of radiation exposure by as much as 89%.[10] It offers several benefits, including preoperative planning and assessment of the brain parenchyma and ventricles.[11]

After workup and confirmation of the diagnosis, treatment recommendations are most consistently for surgical intervention. When discussing surgery with the family, an intraoperative team approach between neurosurgery and plastic surgery is presented. Because intervention is limited to the calvarium external to the dura, the risk of neural parenchymal injury is low. However, it is important to explain the potential, although unlikely, for life-threatening bleeding, especially if there is iatrogenic injury to a dural sinus. Significantly more common is the need for perioperative blood transfusion because small children are unable to tolerate intraoperative losses owing to a smaller starting blood pool than adults. Thus, nearly all children require at least intraoperative blood transfusion and this procedure should also be discussed when consenting for surgery. Many families prefer directed blood donation, which should also be offered at this time.

SAGITTAL CRANIOSYNOSTOSIS

Sagittal craniosynostosis is the most common form of craniosynostosis and represents 45% of cases.[12] Premature fusion of the sagittal suture restricts widening of the calvarium, resulting in compensatory excessive anterior-posterior (AP) lengthening, frontal bossing, and occipital bulleting.[2,9] This growth pattern is termed scaphocephaly owing to the resultant "boat-shaped" deformity it produces (**Fig. 2**).

Owing to the midline nature of the defect, it lends itself well to a variety of surgical treatments, including early intervention. Early intervention is accomplished through sagittal suturectomy and may be performed either in a traditional open or endoscopic-assisted fashion, which affords a minimally invasive approach. Other options include more extensive strip craniectomies in combination with AP shortening or total vault remodeling. All of these procedures are usually combined with parietotemporal barrel staving to facilitate skull widening into a more natural round head shape.[13,14]

As mentioned, early intervention requires it be performed by 3 to 4 months of age. Although surgery is performed earlier in the child's life, the desired final outcome requires a period of postoperative helmet therapy for the ensuing 3 to 6 months. This duration of therapy correlates with the known period of exponential brain growth, which causes expansion of the calvarium. During this time, AP growth is restricted by the rigid helmet, allowing lateral widening with selective subtraction of the padding material within the helmet. Failure to perform surgical intervention by this time results in suboptimal outcomes owing to comparative slowed brain growth and a thickened calvarium.

When performed in a minimally invasive fashion, 2 limited parallel coronal incisions are made just

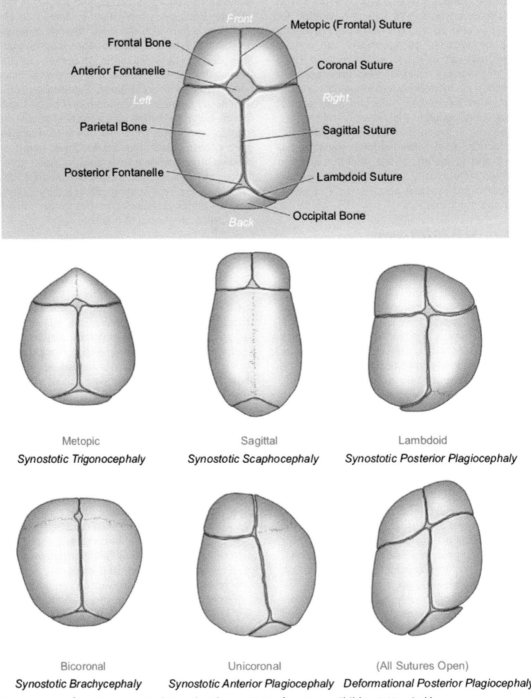

Fig. 1. Types of craniosynostosis. (Printed with permission from Texas Children's Hospital.)

posterior to the anterior fontanel and 2 to 3 cm anterior to the lambda. The scalp is then elevated off the calvarium in a subgaleal plane. A 4- to 5-cm strip of bone is removed to include the entire sagittal suture. Bilateral anterior and posterior lateral wedge osteotomies are then made down to the level of the squamosal suture to facilitate biparietal widening and reshaping with future helmet therapy (**Fig. 3**). The endoscope is used when performing the osteotomies to guide the

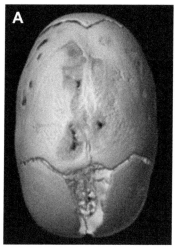
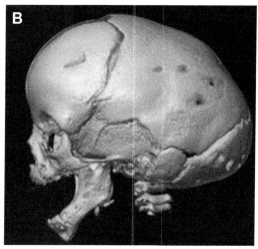

Fig. 2. Three-dimensional computed tomography reconstruction of a sagittal craniosynostosis. (*A*) Bird's eye view (forehead oriented down) demonstrating prematurely fused sagittal suture with associated parietooccipital narrowing. (*B*) Lateral view demonstrating classic scaphocephaly with associated occipital bulleting.

cutting vector and ensure dural protection. Fastidious hemostasis is ensured after copious irrigation before incision closure because no drains are placed.

In recent years, some have advocated for intermediate timed (usually between 3 and 8 months of age) intervention using spring assistance.[15,16] The

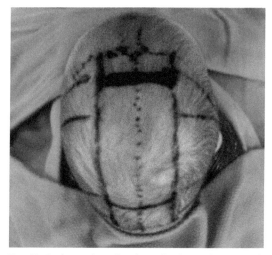

Fig. 3. Endoscopic-assisted sagittal craniosynostosis repair design. Vertex view with the patient in the prone position of planned incisions (*medial solid coronal lines*), sagittal strip craniectomy (*medial solid sagittal lines*), and closing wedge osteotomies (*lateral solid lines*). The sagittal, coronal, and lambdoid sutures are shown as *dotted lines*. Note the position of the anterior (*down*) and posterior (*up*) incisions with respect to the anterior fontanelle and lambda respectively.

spring facilitates biparietal vault widening after the window of exponential brain growth used during molding helmet therapy has closed. This intervention can be performed in a minimally invasive fashion similar to endoscopic assisted strip craniectomy. Consequently, it offers the associated benefit of a decreased duration of hospital stay and lower transfusion requirement.[17,18] However, it does require a second surgery for spring device removal. There also remains controversy over the amount of spring force and number of devices required to obtain equivalent results to open cranial vault remodeling. This in addition to the requisite dual procedures associated with this treatment have resulted in slow adoption of the technique, including at our institution. Further research is ongoing to perfect the technique as well as development of a resorbable device that would eliminate the need for a second procedure.

Open repair is deferred until 6 months of age to allow adequate development for the child to more safely tolerate the associated surgical stress of the procedure. The thinner and more malleable cranial bones at this age also facilitate easier contouring of the parietal skull, correction of occipital bulleting, and AP shortening without total vault remodeling compared with the older child. The senior author favors a modified pi technique in which the child is placed in a prone position. Ensuring the airway and eyes are protected during this maneuver is of paramount importance. Consequently, the endotracheal tube is secured with a circumandibular suture while still in the supine position and face padded with an adhesive foam ring to avoid pressure on the eyes. A bicoronal sawtooth shaped incision is then planned within the hair bearing scalp over the vertex of the skull (**Fig. 4**). Either a thin strip of hair or the entire head is then shaved at the parents' request and the scalp widely infiltrated with epinephrine containing local anesthesia. Dissection is carried down to the level of the periosteum, which is left intact over the calvarium. Osteotomies are then designed to remove a 2- to 3-cm strip of bone including the entire sagittal suture. Note that this is significantly narrower than the strip removed with early intervention. Osteotomies both anterior and posterior to the coronal and lambdoid sutures are made to "float" the sutures in addition to several lateral barrel stave osteotomies inferiorly to the level of the squamosal suture (**Fig. 5**). This facilitates contouring of the temporal, parietal, and occipital regions. In severely elongated heads AP shortening is achieved through bilateral posteriorly based lateral closing wedge osteotomies. The sagittal strip is shortened accordingly (usually 1–2 cm) and then inset with PDS suspension sutures for neural protection. A single 10F closed suction drain is left exiting behind the ear, which allows for egress of reactive fluid accumulation from the more extensive dissection compared with early intervention.

In the absence of intraoperative complications or confounding comorbid conditions, all children are admitted to the floor postoperatively. Early intervention children are monitored overnight and most frequently discharged the following morning if feeding well and normocemic. They are then fitted with their molding helmet, which is applied after 1 week to allow the scalp incisions to heal. Later intervention children stay a minimum of 2 nights. Their drain is removed routinely on the second postoperative day, regardless of output, which we have found may be safely done without adverse sequelae. They are most frequently able to be discharged at this time unless suffering from periorbital edema preventing eye opening, which is rare with this operation.

Children undergoing helmet therapy are seen monthly until completion of therapy (**Fig. 6**). All children are followed at 3-, 6-, and 12-month intervals thereafter until the age of 6. During these visits, symptoms of recurrent synostosis are screened including headache, nausea, disordered sleep, abnormal neurodevelopment, and yearly dilated eye examinations to evaluate for papilledema. Residual soft spots, representing nonreossified areas of the skull, are also noted. Even if present, they rarely require intervention unless larger than 2 cm^2.

CORONAL CRANIOSYNOSTOSIS

Coronal craniosynostosis is the second most common form of craniosynostosis accounting for approximately 25% cases, the vast majority of which are unicoronal.[12] Unicoronal cases are characterized by ipsilateral flattening of the forehead on the synostotic side and bossin of the

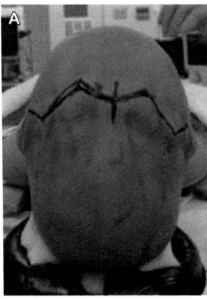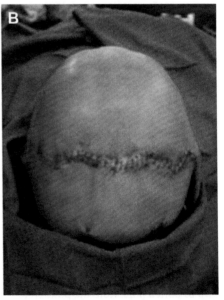

Fig. 4. Open sagittal craniosynostosis repair. (*A*) Vertex view of a 6-month-old sagittal craniosynostosis patient in the prone position with planned bicoronal saw tooth incision. (*B*) Immediate on table postoperative result after cranial vault remodeling with anteroposterior shortening using a modified Pi technique.

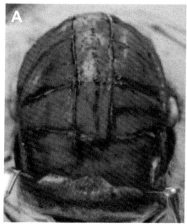
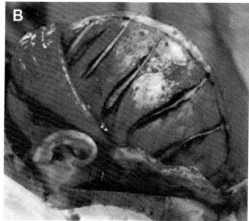

Fig. 5. Modified Pi osteotomy design. (*A*) Vertex and (*B*) right lateral views of a 6-month-old sagittal craniosynostosis patient in the prone position with planned osteotomy pattern. Note the parietotemporal barrel stave osteotomies extend inferiorly to the squamosal suture. These coronal osteotomies are also made anterior and posterior to the coronal and lambdoid sutures, allowing them to "float" in the newly remodeled calvarium.

contralateral frontoparietal skull, known as anterior deformational plagiocephaly. The resultant restriction of forehead growth is believed to create compensatory pressure on the maxilla by the ipsilateral temporal lobe, resulting in the rotation of the midface, commonly known as the facial twist. Consequently, there is forward displacement of the ipsilateral zygoma and deviation of the nasal tip to the contralateral side (**Fig. 7**).[2] In contrast, bilateral coronal craniosynostosis creates uniform AP growth restriction and shortening with bitemporal widening, referred to as brachycephaly. Instead of the characteristic facial twist observed in unilateral cases, there is compensatory craniocaudal skull elongation, referred to as turricephaly (**Fig. 8**).[9]

Correction of either unicoronal or bicoronal deformity is focused on not only the forehead, but also the superolateral orbits. This correction is accomplished through removal of the frontal bones and orbital bandeau for recontouring and repositioning, known as frontoorbital advancement. This procedure requires a fairly extensive dissection extending from the vertex of the scalp posteriorly to the frontonasal suture anteriorly and laterally to the squamosal and zygomaticofrontal sutures, respectively. Consequently, intervention is deferred to approximately 10 to 12 months of age to be performed in an open fashion.

Similar to open sagittal craniosynostosis repair, a bicoronal sawtooth incision is made within the

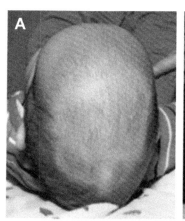
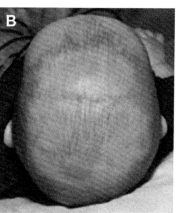
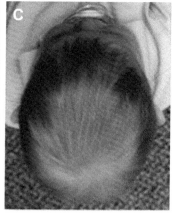

Fig. 6. Endoscopic-assisted sagittal craniosynostosis repair results. (*A*) Birds eye view of a 3-month-old child with sagittal craniosynostosis and scaphocephaly. (*B*) The 6-week postoperative result after endoscopic-assisted sagittal strip craniectomy with bilateral parietal closing wedge osteotomies and molding helmet therapy. (*C*) The 6-month postoperative result after cessation of helmet therapy.

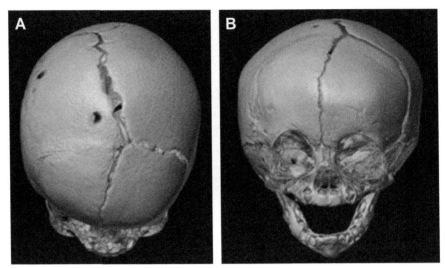

Fig. 7. Three-dimensional computed tomography reconstruction of right unicoronal craniosynostosis. (*A*) Bird's eye view demonstrating ipsilateral forehead flattening and anterior displacement of the zygoma with contralateral forehead bossing. (*B*) Anterior view demonstrating superolateral distortion of the ipsilateral orbit and nasomaxillary deviation toward the contralateral side, "facial twist."

hair-bearing scalp. However, the patient is in a supine position to facilitate access to the forehead and orbital bandeau. Additionally, dissection is carried in a subperiosteal plane to the limits described previously. A bifrontal craniotomy is then performed leaving approximately 17 mm of bone stock above the superior orbital rim to provide adequate rigidity of the orbital bandeau to be removed later. The bifrontal craniotomy may be performed in either 1 or 2 pieces depending on the craniofacial and neurosurgeon preference and comfort level working over the sagittal sinus.

The orbital bandeau is then removed en bloc using a C-shaped osteotomy through the zygoma and orbital roof. In unicoronal cases, additional temporal bone is often included on the affected side to minimize a zygomaticofrontal suture boney step off after it is re-inset. Recontouring of the bandeau requires focal weakening at the glabella to allow forward rotation of the affected side into a symmetric curve. This maneuver invariably widens the lateral temporal wing of the affected side, which is then narrowed through a closing wedge osteotomy on the inner table of the lateral

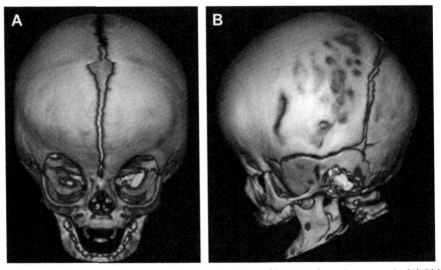

Fig. 8. Three-dimensional computed tomography reconstruction of bicoronal craniosynostosis. (*A*) Oblique bird's eye view demonstrating bitemporal widening. (*B*) Left lateral view demonstrating the tall flattened forehead seen in turribrachycephaly.

orbital wall. The curve of the newly contoured bandeau is stabilized with absorbable plates on the inner table. In select cases, onlay bone grafts may be placed to augment brow projection on the affected side. These are easily obtained from the frontal craniotomy ex vivo or exposed parietal bone in vivo. Additionally, inner table bone shavings are harvested from the frontal craniotomy to fill any residual large bony gaps.

The bandeau is then re-inset onto the skull in a newly advanced and rotated position to optimize brow position. This is secured to the pterion with absorbable plates and the nasofrontal suture with wire. The frontal bones are then recontoured to correct the flattened synostotic side and match the newly contoured bandeau. This is sometimes facilitated by splitting the frontal bones into 2 pieces if removed as a single unit originally. Appropriate orientation and position of the frontal bones is then chosen to optimize forehead shape, which may favor a switch cranioplasty. The frontal bones are then inset with multiple PDS sutures placed through small wire pass holes to the bandeau. In general, overcorrection is favored to accommodate minor relapse and future growth.

Additional contouring of the restricted parietal bones is achieved with outfracture of the posteriorly based barrel stave osteotomies. The temporal bony gaps created by the advancement are filled with the previously mentioned inner table shavings bone graft. Lateral canthoplasties are also performed to appropriately position the canthus as they are stripped with the initial dissection. The scalp is then closed over a subgaleal drain.

It is important to note and counsel the family that the facial twist seen in unicoronal craniosynostosis is not fully corrected with this procedure. Furthermore, no other procedure has been found to fully and consistently correct the deformity. However, it seems that earlier intervention stops propagation of the deformity, which is also partially disguised by future facial growth (**Fig. 9**).[19,20]

The procedure is modified in bicoronal cases so that lateral closing wedge osteotomies are performed along the inner table of both lateral orbital walls to narrow the bitemporal width. Although recontouring of the glabella is usually not necessary in these cases, a similar advancement and rotation is still used to optimize brow position when re-insetting the bandeau (**Fig. 10**).

The postoperative course is similar to the sagittal craniosynostosis children. However, expected hospital stay is usually 3 to 5 days owing to inevitable periorbital swelling, preventing eye opening, which we require to be resolved in at least 1 eye before discharge.

METOPIC CRANIOSYNOSTOSIS

Metopic craniosynostosis is the third most common form of craniosynostosis, accounting for approximately 20% of cases. Because the metopic suture is the first to fuse, within the first 6 to 12 months of life, differentiating between a normal overriding suture ridge and pathologic synostosis is imperative.[21] Metopic craniosynostosis results from suture fusion either in utero or shortly after birth, which produces pathognomonic trigoncephaly. This is characterized by a triangular-shaped forehead with associated bitemporal narrowing and hypotelorism (**Fig. 11**). In contrast, these features are absent in benign metopic ridging and the ridge is a normal variant created by an overriding suture after normal fusion several months after birth.

Only metopic craniosynostosis requires surgical intervention, which is amenable to both early and late intervention. Early intervention is usually performed at 3 months of age through a minimally invasive endoscopic approach. A limited V-shaped incision is made behind the hairline of the anterior scalp in midline. Subgaleal dissection is then carried inferiorly to the level of the nasofrontal suture and posteriorly to the anterior fontanel. A wedged strip suturectomy is then performed to include the metopic suture. Oblique barrel stave osteotomies are also performed laterally to allow recontouring of the frontal bones from the anterior fontanel to the superior orbital rim (**Fig. 12**). This incision is closed without a drain and the postoperative course is similar to that of the endoscopic-assisted sagittal suturectomy patients, including a course of molding helmet therapy (**Fig. 13**).

Late intervention is performed at 10 to 12 months of age and is similar to the technique described in the coronal craniosynostosis section via frontoorbital advancement. However, there are some key differences between the 2 procedures. Although exposure and craniotomies are performed in an identical fashion, different considerations are given to remodeling the bandeau. Specifically, the bandeau requires glabellar widening to correct hypotelorism. This is accomplished by splitting the bandeau ex-vivo and placement of an 8 to 10 mm interposition bone graft obtained from the exposed parietal bone. The new bandeau construct is then secured and re-inset on the skull with absorbable plates in a similar fashion to that described in the coronal craniosynostosis repair to optimize brow position. The frontal bones are also similarly replaced, posteriorly based parietal barrel stave osteotomies performed, and large bony gaps filled with harvested inner table bone

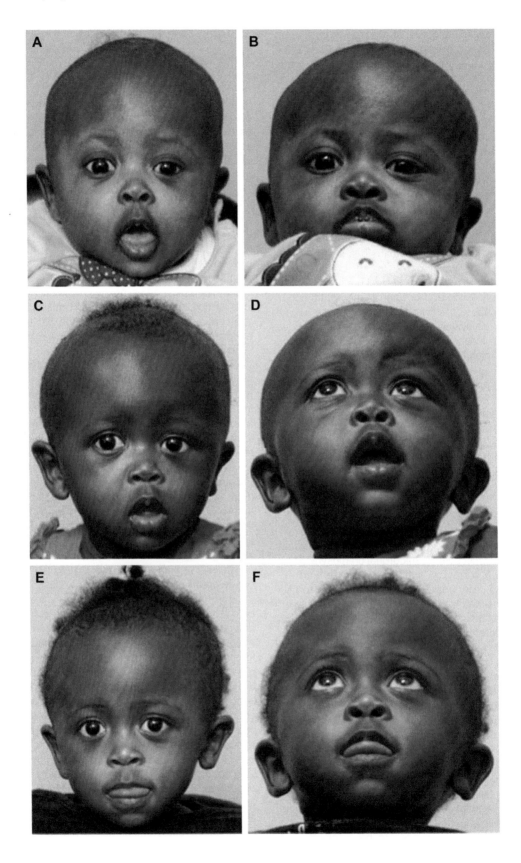

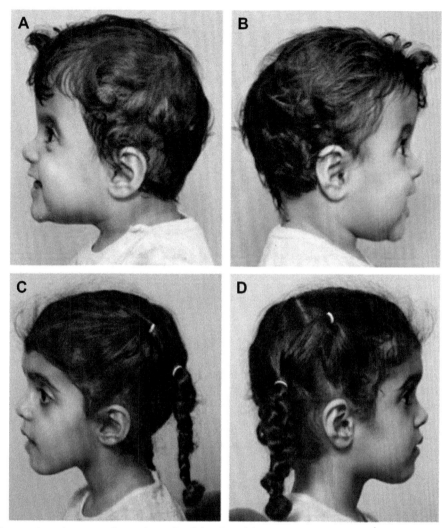

Fig. 10. Bicoronal craniosynostosis repair results. (*A*) Left and (*B*) right lateral preoperative views of a 12-month-old bicoronal craniosynostosis patient. Note the turribrachycephaly with a tall, broad, and flattened forehead. (*C*) Left and (*D*) right 2-year postoperative views after frontoorbital advancement with improved forehead shape.

graft shavings (**Fig. 14**). The postoperative course is identical for both frontoorbital advancement procedures (**Fig. 15**).

LAMBDOID CRANIOSYNOSTOSIS

Lambdoid craniosynostosis is rare, accounting for less than 5% of all cases.[9] Most frequently presenting in unilateral form, the resultant deformity produces bossing of the ipsilateral mastoid process and downward displacement of the cranial base on the affected side creating an apparent tilt. There is also compensatory bossing of the contralateral parietal skull (**Fig. 16**). Differentiating between lambdoid craniosynostosis and positional plagiocephaly is additionally aided by

Fig. 9. Unicoronal craniosynostosis repair results. (*A*) Preoperative frontal and (*B*) worm's eye views of a 3-month-old right unicoronal craniosynostosis patient. Note the right orbital and brow superolateral distortion with forehead flattening, contralateral bossing, and mild nasomaxillary deviation toward the left. Patient underwent frontoorbital advancement at 10 months of age. (*C*, *D*) The 2-week postoperative results showing improved forehead shape and brow position with planned overcorrection. (*E*, *F*) Durable results at 8 months postoperatively without progression of the facial "twist" deformity.

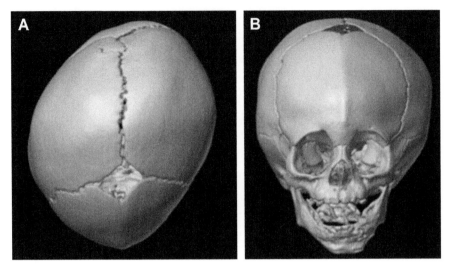

Fig. 11. Three-dimensional computed tomography reconstruction of metopic craniosynostosis. (*A*) Bird's eye view (*forehead oriented down*) demonstrating trigoncephaly. Note the superimposed right positional plagiocephaly. (*B*) Anterior view demonstrating bitemporal narrowing and hypotelorism.

looking the position of the ear. Classically, it has been taught that positional plagiocephaly results in anterior displacement and lambdoid craniosynostosis in posterior displacement of the ear. However, this has been shown to be an unreliable predictor. However, owing to the downward tilt of the cranial base on the affected side, the entire ear is subsequently inferiorly displaced. These 2 findings have proven significantly more reliable in identifying children with surgically correctable synostosis.[22]

Surgical correction requires remodeling of the posterior vault. Although the deformity has been adequately treated with strip craniectomy in some patients, including in an early intervention endoscopic assisted fashion, we have found

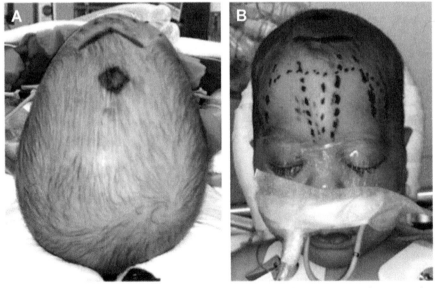

Fig. 12. Endoscopic-assisted metopic craniosynostosis repair design. (*A*) Vertex view of a 3-month-old metopic craniosynostosis patient demonstrating a V-shaped posttrichal incision and anterior fontanelle. (*B*) Anterior view of planned wedge-shaped midline strip craniectomy pattern to include the fused metopic suture and lateral barrel stave osteotomies. Note these lines extend to the anterior fontanelle.

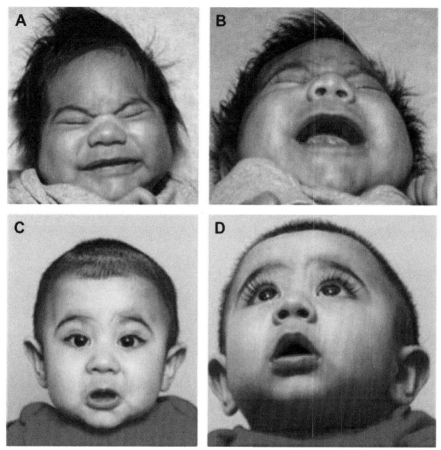

Fig. 13. Endoscopic-assisted metopic craniosynostosis repair results. (*A*) Frontal and (*B*) worm's eye preoperative views of a 3-month-old metopic craniosynostosis patient. Note the marked trigoncephaly and bitemporal narrowing. (*C, D*) The 6-month postoperative results at the conclusion of helmet therapy showing restoration of bitemporal width and improved forehead shape.

more reliable results are obtained through open posterior vault remodeling approximately 6 months of age. This technique involves prone positioning and surgical access similar to the open approach described in the sagittal craniosynostosis section.

The posterior parietal and occipital bones are then removed, taking care to avoid injury to the torcula. If removed en bloc, it is then divided and contoured ex vivo. The hallmark of the operation is switching the right and left newly contoured occipital bones when placed back on the skull. This switch cranioplasty provides increased volume to the affected side, which is then secured with absorbable plates. Additional parietal barrel staving of the bossed unaffected side is added as necessary to create a normal contour. The scalp is closed over a closed suction drain with a similar postoperative course to the modified pi patient described in the sagittal craniosynostosis section.

This technique for open posterior vault remodeling through switch cranioplasty is very effective at correcting the flattened occiput on the affected side and contralateral parietal bossing. However, it does not address the ipsilateral mastoid bossing or cranial base tilt, and no adjuvant procedure has been found to reliably and safely correct the abnormality. However, similar to the facial twist seen with unicoronal craniosynostosis, earlier intervention does seem to stop progression of the deformity (**Fig. 17**).

COMPLICATIONS AND OUTCOMES

Major complications are rare after cranial vault remodeling and classified as either early or late.[23] Acute complications of cranial vault remodeling include bleeding, infection, cerebrospinal fluid leak, meningitis, and stroke, which can all be potentially life threatening. Owing to the risk of significant bleeding, it is important to have blood readily available with sufficient intravenous access during surgery in the event this complication is encountered.

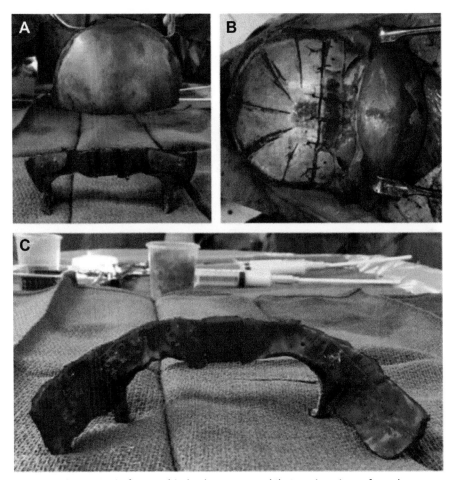

Fig. 14. Metopic craniosynostosis frontoorbital advancement. (*A*) Anterior view of newly contoured orbital bandeau in relation to noncontoured frontal bones. Note the increased bitemporal diameter achieved and correction of hypoteleroism with the interposed parietal bone graft. Brow position is augmented with bilateral onlay bone grafts as well. (*B*) Anterior view bandeau and frontal bones re-inset on the skull after recontouring to maximize forehead width and brow position. (*C*) Posterior view of contoured bandeau. Note the closing wedge osteotomies made at the lateral orbital wall to facilitate contouring of the temporal bones. Inner table bone shavings used to fill large temporoparietal bony defects are seen in the specimen cup at the top of the photo.

Potentially, and equally devastating, is the migration of an air embolus through a dural sinus and should be monitored for with a precordial Doppler ultrasound examination intraoperatively. Dural tears without underlying sinus injury are much more common and should be repaired intraoperatively if identified. If a cerebrospinal fluid leak is identified or suspected postoperatively, it is usually self-limiting with minor interventions such as removing suction from overlying drains. Persistent leak requires lumbar drain placement or surgical exploration and repair. Cases of meningitis are exceedingly uncommon, but usually seen in the setting of a cerebrospinal fluid leak or open communication with the nasal cavity and require prompt antibiotic treatment and intervention to repair the inciting etiology. Overall, the mortality rate of from treatment of craniosynostosis is well below 1%.

Late complications include contour irregularities and failure of reossification, both of which can result in the need for reoperation. Failure of reossification is estimated to be between 5% and 20%, with a positive correlation with increased age at time of repair. In general, only defects of greater than 2 cm^2 are recommended for repair. Some "lumpy bumpy" contour irregularity is to be expected after repair, and usually improves with time. More significant contour irregularities are often treated with PEEK cranioplasty if bothersome to the patient or family, though should be

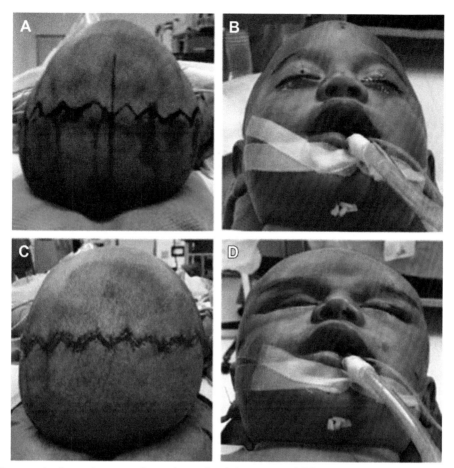

Fig. 15. Open metopic craniosynostosis repair results. (*A*) Vertex and (*B*) worm's eye preoperative views of a 12-month-old metopic craniosynostosis patient. Note the trigoncephaly and hypotelorism. (*C, D*) Immediate on-table postoperative result after frontoorbital advancement. Note the improved forehead shape, brow position, and orbital position. Overcorrection is favored to allow for future growth and minor relapse.

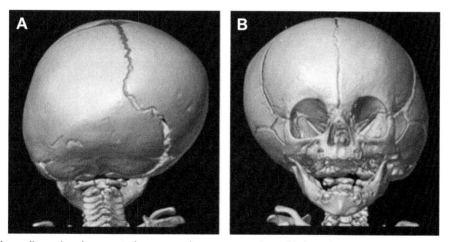

Fig. 16. Three-dimensional computed tomography reconstruction of left unilateral lambdoid craniosynostosis. (*A*) Posterior view of deformational plagiocephaly from a prematurely fused left lambdoid suture. Note the ipsilateral mastoid and contralateral parietal bossing with associated downward tilt of the cranial base toward the affected side. (*B*) Ipsilateral mastoid and contralateral parietal bossing is readily apparent on the anterior view.

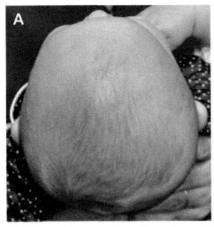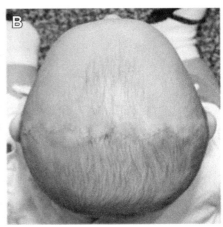

Fig. 17. Lambdoid craniosynostosis repair results. (*A*) Vertex view of a 6-month-old left unilateral lambdoid cra-niosynostosis patient. Note the left deformational plagiocephaly and posteriorly displaced ear. (*B*) Early 2-week postoperative result after switch cranioplasty with improved head shape and ear position.

deferred until the age of 6 to minimize subsequent changes from head growth.

SUMMARY

Abnormal head shape continues to be a common reason for referral to the craniofacial surgeon. An increasing percentage of referrals are now sec-ondary to underlying craniosynostosis thanks to improved education and methods of detection by referring providers. Nonsyndromic craniosynosto-sis may be safely and reliably corrected through the multiple techniques discussed. However, future research is needed to continue to refine our surgical techniques into increasingly minimally invasive methods, which decrease operative risk. Additionally, further investigation is warranted into the underlying genetic causes of craniosynos-tosis, which may eventually be manipulated to pro-vide nonoperative treatment options to the developing synostotic child.

REFERENCES

1. Mawji A, Vollman AR, Hatfield J, et al. The incidence of positional plagiocephaly: a cohort study. Pediat-rics 2013;132(2):298–304.
2. Persing JA. MOC-PS(SM) CME article: management considerations in the treatment of craniosynostosis. Plast Reconstr Surg 2008;121(4 Suppl):1–11.
3. Hunenko O, Karmacharya J, Ong G, et al. Toward an understanding of nonsyndromic craniosynostosis: altered patterns of TGF-beta receptor and FGF re-ceptor expression induced by intrauterine head constraint. Ann Plast Surg 2001;46(5):546–53 [dis-cussion: 553–4].
4. Boyadjiev SA, International Craniosynostosis Con-sortium. Genetic analysis of non-syndromic craniosynostosis. Orthod Craniofac Res 2007; 10(3):129–37.
5. Buchanan EP, Xue Y, Xue AS, et al. Multidisciplinary care of craniosynostosis. J Multidiscip Healthc 2017; 10:263–70.
6. Thompson DN, Harkness W, Jones B, et al. Subdural intracranial pressure monitoring in craniosynostosis: its role in surgical management. Childs Nerv Syst 1995;11(5):269–75.
7. Kapp-Simon KA, Speltz ML, Cunningham ML, et al. Neurodevelopment of children with single suture craniosynostosis: a review. Childs Nerv Syst 2007; 23(3):269–81.
8. Persing JA, Jane JA, Shaffrey M. Virchow and the path-ogenesis of craniosynostosis: a translation of his orig-inal work. Plast Reconstr Surg 1989;83(4):738–42.
9. Mathes SJ, Hentz VR. Plastic surgery, vol. 4. Phila-delphia: Saunders Elsevier; 2006.
10. Harshbarger R, Kelley P, Leake D, et al. Low dose craniofacial CT/rapid access MRI protocol in cranio-synostosis patients: decreased radiation exposure and cost savings. Plast Reconstr Surg 2010;126:4–5.
11. Fearon JA, Singh DJ, Beals SP, et al. The diagnosis and treatment of single-sutural synostoses: are computed tomographic scans necessary? Plast Re-constr Surg 2007;120(5):1327–31.
12. Kolar JC. An epidemiological study of nonsyndromal craniosynostoses. J Craniofac Surg 2011;22(1):47–9.
13. Fearon JA, McLaughlin EB, Kolar JC. Sagittal cranio-synostosis: surgical outcomes and long-term growth. Plast Reconstr Surg 2006;117(2):532–41.
14. Cohen SR, Pryor L, Mittermiller PA, et al. Nonsyn-dromic craniosynostosis: current treatment options. Plast Surg Nurs 2008;28(2):79–91.
15. David LR, Plikaitis CM, Couture D, et al. Outcome analysis of our first 75 spring-assisted surgeries for scaphocephaly. J Craniofac Surg 2010;21(1):3–9.

16. David LR, Proffer P, Hurst WJ, et al. Spring-mediated cranial reshaping for craniosynostosis. J Craniofac Surg 2004;15(5):810–6 [discussion: 817–8].

17. Gerety PA, Basta MN, Fischer JP, et al. Operative management of nonsyndromic sagittal synostosis: a head-to-head meta-analysis of outcomes comparing 3 techniques. J Craniofac Surg 2015; 26(4):1251–7.

18. Sun J, Ter Maaten NS, Mazzaferro DM, et al. Spring-mediated cranioplasty in sagittal synostosis: does age at placement affect expansion? J Craniofac Surg 2018;29(3):632–5.

19. Miri S, Mittermiller P, Buchanan EP, et al. Facial twist (asymmetry) in isolated unilateral coronal synostosis: does premature facial suture fusion play a role? J Craniofac Surg 2015;26(3):655–7.

20. Mundinger GS, Skladman R, Wenger T, et al. Defining and correcting asymmetry in isolated unilateral frontosphenoidal synostosis: differences in orbital shape, facial scoliosis, and skullbase twist compared to unilateral coronal synostosis. J Craniofac Surg 2018;29(1):29–35.

21. Weinzweig J, Kirschner RE, Farley A, et al. Metopic synostosis: defining the temporal sequence of normal suture fusion and differentiating it from synostosis on the basis of computed tomography images. Plast Reconstr Surg 2003;112(5):1211–8.

22. Ploplys EA, Hopper RA, Muzaffar AR, et al. Comparison of computed tomographic imaging measurements with clinical findings in children with unilateral lambdoid synostosis. Plast Reconstr Surg 2009;123(1):300–9.

23. Czerwinski M, Hopper RA, Gruss J, et al. Major morbidity and mortality rates in craniofacial surgery: an analysis of 8101 major procedures. Plast Reconstr Surg 2010;126(1):181–6.

Syndromic Craniosynostosis

Rajendra Sawh-Martinez, MD, MHS[a], Derek M. Steinbacher, DMD, MD[b],*

KEYWORDS

- Craniofacial syndromes • Craniosynostosis • FGFR • Apert • Crouzon • Muenke • Pfeiffer
- Saethre-Chotzen

KEY POINTS

- Complex multisuture craniosynostosis with varying comorbidities is a hallmark of syndromic craniosynostosis.
- Understanding of the genetic and molecular underpinnings of this array of disorders continues to evolve.
- Individualized, multidisciplinary team-based clinical approaches are required for the care of affected patients.
- Surgical approaches must be tailored to the individual patient deformities, psychosocial family tolerance of multistaged surgical interventions, and developmental prognosis.

INTRODUCTION

Syndromic craniosynostosis encompasses an array of diagnoses and genetic mutations that affect the cranial vault, with additional anomalies in embryologically distinct anatomic sites (**Figs. 1 and 2**). Craniosynostosis refers to the premature fusion of cranial sutures, with inhibition of perpendicular cranial bone growth. These premature fusions may affect a single cranial suture or present in varied patterns of multisuture closure combinations. This premature fusion may occur both as part of a syndrome or in isolation. There are myriad identified genetic mutations that have been linked, with well-described syndromes that commonly present with craniosynostosis.[1–4] These diagnoses have a range of clinical presentations related to the underlying syndromes, and the associated cranial suture fusions have their own spectrum of presentation,

both of which are linked to the genetic underpinnings of disease. Generally, patients affected by these syndromic craniosynostosis are believed to have multisuture involvement with significant potential for restricted brain growth, increased intracranial pressure (ICP), and facial dysmorphisms in the setting of a spectrum of additional anatomic anomalies.[1,5,6] For an individually affected patient, however, their presentation can vary from mild to very severe anatomic anomalies, mandating an individualized, multispecialty approach to the successful treatment of each patient. Currently, more than 180 syndromes are known to be associated with craniosynostosis.[7] Various reviews detail the commonly presented craniosynostosis syndromes and their characteristics.[1,2,6,8,9] The purpose of this article is to provide readers with a framework to understand how to best approach the diagnosis, management, and surgical

The authors have nothing to disclose.
[a] Section of Plastic and Reconstructive Surgery, Department of Surgery, Yale University, 330 Cedar Street, Boardman Building, 3rd Floor, New Haven, CT 06511, USA; [b] Section of Plastic and Reconstructive Surgery, Oral and Maxillofacial Surgery, Department of Surgery, Yale-New Haven Hospital, Yale University, 330 Cedar Street, Boardman Building, 3rd Floor, New Haven, CT 06511, USA
* Corresponding author.
E-mail address: Derek.Steinbacher@yale.edu

Clin Plastic Surg 46 (2019) 141–155
https://doi.org/10.1016/j.cps.2018.11.009

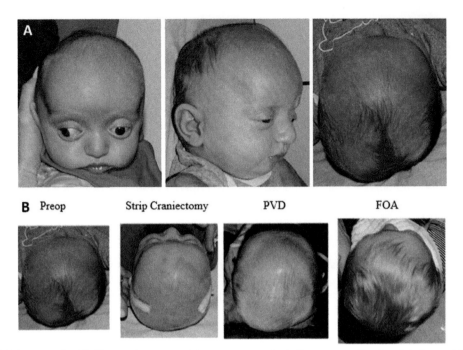

Fig. 1. (*A*) Preoperative Pfeiffer syndrome—multisuture synostosis. *Left* - preoperative frontal view, *middle* - oblique view, *right* - Birds eye view. (*B*) Staged surgical correction. Sequential cranial re-shaping. *First* panel demonstrates preoperative position. *Second* panel demonstrates position after strip craniectomy of coronal sutures. *Third* demonstrates position after posterior vault distraction. *Final* panel demonstrates cranial position after frontoorbital advancement and the final post operative cranial shape. FOA, frontoorbital advancement; Preop, preoperative view; PVD, posterior vault distraction.

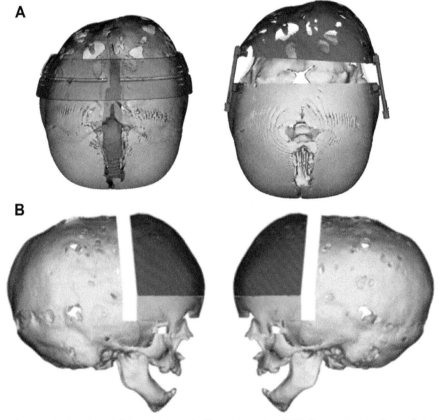

Fig. 2. Virtual surgical planning. (*A*) Posterior vault distraction plan (*left*) demonstrates planned osteotomy site for planned posterior vault distraction and anticipated expansion (*right*) Asymmetric final expansion plan to account for preoperative asymmetry. (*B*) Fronto-orbital advancement, frontal craniotomy *Left* and *right* views of planned position after frontoorbital advancement.

correction options of the craniofacial anomalies that occur in any form and variant of syndromic craniosynostosis.

HISTORICAL PERSPECTIVE

Cultural references and archeological discoveries of varying head shape morphologies can be found in multiple cultures from historical times, dating back to prehistoric times to include the Pleistocene epoch, where the early human ancestors gave way to current *Homo sapiens sapiens* species.[10–13] In antiquity, examples of Egyptian pharaohs, Greek politicians, and indigenous American civilizations are noted to have had representatives and leaders with abnormal head shapes.[12,14,15] Although there were some cultures that revered aberrant cranial morphologies, major craniofacial abnormalities have historically been regarded negatively and with significant prejudice.[16]

Early descriptions of skull shape abnormalities are ascribed to Vesalius, who described oxycephaly in 1543.[17] Written in German, the first description of a fused cranial suture is ascribed to Otto in 1830.[18] Classification of varying skull morphologies was reported by Virchow in 1851 and includes terminology used to this day.[19,20] Early surgical approaches attempting to remove the affected cranial sutures were reported in the nineteenth century.[16,21] These efforts were mired by high mortality rates and limited improvements because regrowth of the affected cranial sutures prevented correction. As techniques evolved, various attempts at increasing osteotomy gaps and arresting bony growth were developed but faced limited success, yielding to a series of described surgical approaches aimed at a more robust cranial remodeling.[22–24]

Surgical approaches to the growing midface was borne out of surgical advancements from approaches to facial trauma during World War I and World War II. The advent of increasingly stable fixation methods provided a quantum leap in surgeons' ability to mobilize and stabilize the craniofacial skeleton.[25–27] Early pioneers in trauma included René Le Fort, who described 3 classic fracture patterns.[28,29] These served as the basis for attempts at osteotomizing and mobilizing the midfacial skeleton in patients with congenital deformities. Paul Tessier developed novel approaches to subperiosteal plane dissections around the orbits and to the anterior skull base, classified rare facial clefts, and offered surgical options for patients with previously limited corrective options.[25,30–39] These advancements and contributions ushered in the modern era of craniofacial surgery.

DIAGNOSIS AND WORK-UP

The correct diagnosis and analysis of the craniosynostosis morphology of an individual with an underlying syndrome are critical. The 5 most common associated syndromes and their genetic mutations include Crouzon syndrome (FGFR2), Apert syndrome (FGFR2), Pfeiffer syndrome (FGFR2 and FGFR1), Muenke syndrome (FGFR3), and Saethre-Chotzen (TWIST1). Key distinguishing associated features, in addition to underlying craniosynostosis, are important to recognize and may point in the direction of a clinical diagnosis:

- Apert syndrome: syndactyly of the hands and feet, high arched palates with midface hypoplasia and developmental delay
- Crouzon syndrome: normal hands/feet, intelligence; midface hypoplasia, beaked nose, and exorbitism
- Pfeiffer syndrome: broad thumbs and long toes with cardiac anomalies
- Saethre-Chotzen syndrome: clinodactyly, beaked nose, and low-set hairline with congenital heart defects
- Muenke syndrome: intellectual disability, deafness and thimble like middle phalanges

Comprehensive Evaluation

A careful examination of the cranial, facial, and limb anatomy often yields an initial classification; however, genetics counseling and analysis together with a nuanced, individualized evaluation of distinct features and characteristics are necessary for specific syndromic characterization (**Table 1**).

There are known mutations that lead to these phenotypes, de novo variants, and a multitude of less common syndromes that may develop craniosynostosis with or without facial, body, and limb dysmorphisms.[1,3,4,40–47] A multidisciplinary team is essential for the adequate care of syndromic craniosynostosis patients. In addition to cranial and facial dysmorphology, key factors to evaluate and document include the following:

- Airway compromise
- Intracerebral anomalies (ie, hydrocephalus and Chiari malformations)
- Cardiac anomalies
- Papilledema (as a proxy for elevated ICP)
- Corneal exposure, related visual loss from severe proptosis
- Clefts of the secondary palate
- Malrotation of the gut

Table 1
Most common craniosynostosis syndromes and associated findings

	Genetic	Cranial	Face	Extremities	Cardiac	Neurocognitive
Aperts	Autosomal dominant or sporadic FGFR2	Tturribrachycephaly (bicoronal synostoses) High forehead, steep, flat and associated with transverse frontal skin furrow Short anterior cranial fossa	Orbits: • Exorbitism • Proptosis • Hypertelorism • Down-slanting palpebral fissure Maxillofacial: • High arched palate • Cleft palate • Hypoplastic midface • Class III • Anterior open bite • Pseudoprognathic mandible Soft tissue • Depressed nasal dorsum • Septal deviation • Facial asymmetry Acne vulgaris	Bilateral symmetric syndactyly of hands and feet Fusion of 2nd/3rd/4th digits, mitt hands Short, broad, radially deviated thumb (radial clinodactyly) Deficient first web space	None	ADHD Developmental delay Intellectual disability
Crouzon	Autosomal dominant or sporadic FGFR2	Bicoronal craniosynostosis, lambdoid suture fusion	Orbits: • Exophthalmos • Hypertelorism • Shallow orbits • Ocular proptosis Maxillofacial: • High arched palate • Midface hypoplasia • Anterior open bite Ears: Low-set ears, ear canal malformations, hearing loss Nose: psittichorhina (beak-like nose)	No involvement	PDA, aortic coarctation	Normal cognition Potential Arnold-Chiari malformation

Muenke	AD or sporadic FGFR3	Coronal suture Craniosynostosis	Orbits: normal Maxillofacial: not involved Ears: hearing loss	Thimble-like middle phalanges	None	Intellectual disability, deafness
Carpenter	AR RAB 23	Coronal ± sagittal synostoses	Hypertelorism, downward-sloping palpebral fissures, epicanthal folds, flat/wide nose with large nostrils, None (high arched, narrow palate)	Short hands/fingers/toes ± syndactyly	TGV, PS	MR in 75% of cases
Saethre-Chotzen	Autosomal dominant or sporadic TWIST1	Acrocephaly (coronal + lambdoid) Usually unicoronal/brachycephaly (can be bicoronal)	Facial asymmetry Low-set hairline Ptosis, hypertelorism, strabismus, epicanthal folds. Beaked nose, nasal septal deviation Cleft palate with high arch	2nd/3rd digit syndactyly Broad thumb/hallux with a valgus deformity Clinodactyly	Congenital heart defects	Usually normal (although mild–moderate MR is reported)
Pfeiffer	Type I—AD FGFR2 Types II, III—sporadic FGFR1	Type I—turribrachycephaly Types II/III—Kleeblattschädel (multisuture synostosis)	Maxillary hypoplasia, proptosis, strabismus, hypertelorism Cleft palate	Broad thumbs (and big toes) Simple syndactyly	ASD, PS Tetralogy of Fallot	Variable (type I normal)

Abbreviations: AD, Autosomal dominant; ADHD, Attention deficit hypersensitivity disorder; AR, Autosomal recessive; ASD, Atrial septal defect; PS, Pulmonary artery stenosis; RAB, Ras like in rat brain; Ras, Superfamily G-protein; TGV, Transposition of great vessels.

- Hearing loss
- Intellectual disability
- Congenital limb anomalies

Although the understanding of grouped features of the common syndromes is a fundamental start in the analysis of a presenting patient, a thorough and individualized examination of the whole patient is essential for optimal patient care. Close collaboration with allied team members guides the proper timing of intervention and coordination of care because these patients face multiple potential procedures and surgical interventions.

Genetic Considerations

Advances in molecular and genetic testing have allowed for the identification of myriad mutations that lead to syndromic manifestations, which include the development of craniosynostosis. Complicating matters in phenotypic expression of genetic aberration is that the same mutation may result in varied disorders, with varied expression profiles, because gene expression is affected by gene penetrance and regulatory mechanisms.[1–4,42,45,48–50] Recent discoveries of novel patterns of genetic inheritance and de novo mutations that lead to craniosynostosis expressions point to that underpinnings of craniosynostosis morphology remain in the dawn of understanding.[42,45] Although patient's clinical presentations continue to be classified into classic eponyms, clinical characterization may no longer provide adequate accuracy as our understanding of the underlying genetic aberrations becomes more sophisticated.

CLINICAL MANAGEMENT

Historically, most cases of syndromic craniosynostosis have been diagnosed in the postnatal period. With technological advances in prenatal testing, 2-D and 3-D ultrasound, MRI, and genetic testing have increased the rates of prenatal diagnosing and screening office visits.[51–56] Important understanding of possible associated features may help guide the recommendation for further prenatal imaging and genetic counseling. Importantly, although ultrasound is not diagnostic for premature cranial suture fusion, it may help to find associated craniofacial anomalies, limb anomalies, central nervous system anomalies, and cardiac and visceral anomalies often associated with a named syndrome.

Concerns for possible craniosynostosis in the prenatal period carry important considerations and complexities to be discussed with expectant parents. Invasive and noninvasive genetic testing

may pinpoint specific genetic changes leading to syndromic manifestations; however, given the variable phenotypic expressions, a genetic diagnosis may not fully elucidate the clinical needs for surgical correction.[1,4,42,44,45,48] Complex inheritance patterns and prevalence of de novo mutations are hallmarks in various forms of syndromic craniosynostosis manifestations.[1,4,45,51,57] Consulting with a genetics counselor is a cornerstone of care for families to understand their child's diagnosis, future family planning, and ongoing understanding of the spectrum of causative mutations and underlying cause of craniofacial malformations.

Prenatal focus on potential expectations and plan for supportive measures may ameliorate stress and anxiety for families (**Table 2**). Key considerations include the possibility that significant discrepancies in cranial morphology may necessitate cesarean section delivery. Findings suggestive of mandibular or midface hypoplasia may in turn lead to the requirement for respiratory support mechanisms or tracheostomy early in life. Later in life, milder forms of mandibular/maxillary hypoplasia my manifest with sleep-disordered breathing, including snoring, hypopnea, and obstructive sleep apnea, potentially requiring surgical intervention. Anatomic limitations on feeding may require limited ability to breastfeed, the use of specialized infant bottles with adjusted nipples, and supportive measures from nasogastric tubes to surgically created gastrostomy tubes for parenteral feeding. Limb anomalies often necessitate

Table 2 Surgical algorithm options for syndromic craniosynostosis	
Under 3 mo	Strip craniectomy if evidence of elevated ICP, multisuture synostosis
6–8 mo	Posterior vault distraction as 1st stage
10–18 mo	Definitive cranial vault correction/fronto-orbital advancement
5–9 y	Le Fort III, Le Fort I distraction osteogenesis (early mixed dentition, aimed at correcting exorbitism, midface hypoplasia)
9–12 y	Le Fort III/monobloc advancement 1 stage (late mixed dentition)
15–20 y	Orthognathic surgery to set occlusion, facial balance

surgical correction, with potentially limited ability for patients to have completely restored normal function. Early referral to support groups may assist families in the transition to care for children with complex, chronic clinical care needs.

Coordination of care for these considerations requires a multidisciplinary team approach, with an individualized evaluation and plan of care. The team must also account for each family's psychosocial considerations and ability to support the patient through complex, multistaged surgical and care considerations. The prenatal period is often an ideal time to address these complexities and allow families to begin planning for care of a child with syndromic craniosynostosis.

Postnatal clinical examination drives the consideration and requirement for definitive imaging modalities and surgical timing. CT is currently the mainstay of definitive imaging in diagnosis of early cranial suture fusion and virtual surgical planning.[41,50,58-60] Novel imaging paradigms include the capture of cranial MRI, using gradient echo parameters that allow for improved distinction of bone–soft tissue interfaces.[61] Current and ongoing clinical studies aimed at optimizing the use of this nonionizing radiation imaging modality point toward a new future clinical standard for confirmation of clinical diagnosis and surgical planning.[61-66] Although often attained by referring physicians, skull radiographs offer limited benefit in diagnosis and expose the patient to ionizing radiation. Prenatal ultrasound accuracy and utility is operator dependent, but in experienced hands 3-D ultrasound may offer insights into associated facial dysmorphology and insight into potentially classic cranial patterns associated with prematurely fused cranial sutures.[51]

SURGICAL MANAGEMENT

For the craniofacial surgeon, precise analysis and evaluation of cranial and facial morphology are central to the providing guidance and surgical options to families. Stereotypic cranial morphologies often relate to underlying cranial suture fusion, precluding the need for confirmatory imaging. For complex cases of multisuture craniosynostosis with potential concurrent aberrant brain development, the following considerations are recommended: Evaluate for increased ICP, assess possible overlying positional plagiocephaly, attain imaging for precise diagnosis and analysis of cranial and intracranial findings, in-depth morphometric analysis, and virtual surgical planning are recommended.[57,58,60,67-70] Current strategies for multisuture syndromic craniosynostosis (focused

on common bicoronal and pansynostosis cases) are based on early interventions (2–4 months of age) with prolonged relief of cranial bone fusion (via posterior vault distraction, strip craniectomy ± springs) where imaging (CT and serial skull radiographs) is a key component in the surgical plan for positioning of implanted device, analysis of ongoing care, evaluation of postoperative result, and planning of future intervention[2,58-60,67,71-78] (**Fig. 3**, see **Table 2**).

Commonly, syndromic synostosis cases present with notable turribrachycephaly and may have craniofacial dysmorphisms despite open or partially open cranial sutures that fuse after 6 months of age. The common need for early correction occurs with multisuture involvement. Concerning potential elevations in ICP and impairment in blood flow are believed to lead to poor neurocognitive outcomes.[1,49,70,72,79] Given the spectrum of disease, surgical approaches are geared toward common patterns in suture pathology. Key features to consider in timing of intervention is the clinical and radiographic evidence of increased ICP. Severe restriction and signs of increased ICP may be evident on imaging with noted findings, which may include luckenschadel (lacunar skull), thumbprinting, or copper-beaten skull appearance, all of which may be signs intracranial pathology. Although these can result from intracranial masses, obstructive hydrocephalus, Chiari malformations, or abnormal collagen development and ossification, they may be evident in cases of craniosynostosis. Direct measuring and normal values of ICP are controversial and ill-defined in pediatric and neonatal populations.[80-82] Nonetheless, prevailing standard of care is aimed at relieving the significant growth restriction and cranial deformity that occur with multisuture synostosis. Additionally, development of midface hypoplasia and facial growth restriction often lead to stereotypic facial dysmorphologies that may include exorbitism, maxillary hypoplasia, short noses, hypotelorism, and a narrow high arched palate that require surgical intervention later in childhood.

Although debate remains on the ideal timing for surgical intervention, early intervention for multisuture involvement is believed to lower the impact of increased ICP and curtail the impact of craniofacial dysmorphisms on brain growth and development.[2,58,75,77,83,84] Surgery deferred to later time points allows for increased stability in bony correction and potentially less need for additional or revisionary procedures and may be appropriate for 1 or 2 suture

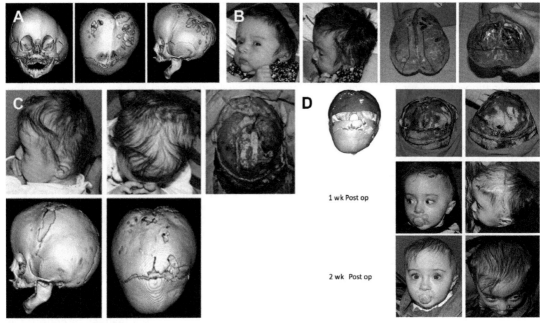

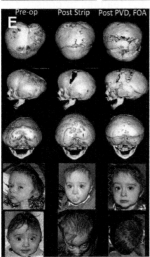

Fig. 3. Management of multisuture synostosis. Recommended surgical timing for cases with evidence of increased intracranial pressure, restricted cranial growth. Strip craniectomy (4–8 wk), PVD (6–8 mo), FOA, cranioplasty (8–10 mo): (*A*) multisuture synostosis (metopic, sagittal, and Kleeblattschadel (multisuture synostosis unilateral coronal) CT scan (*Left* - frontal view, middle - bird's eye view, *right* - lateral view) and (*B*) clinical pictures (*first panel* oblique view, *second panel* lateral view) and 3-D printed skull model (3rd panel bird's eye view, 4th panel posterior view) of patient with FGFR 3 mutation without associated named syndromic features. (*C*) Postoperative photographs, post strip-craniectomy (*left* panel lateral view, *middle* panel Birds eye view, and *right* panel with intraoperative picture), and postoperative CT scan demonstrating refusion of sutures in bottom panels (*bottom left* - lateral view, *bottom right* bird's eye view). (*D*) VSP for PVD, *Top left* panel with CT scan demonstrating final post-distraction desired position, to *middle* panel with bird's eye view of distractor placement, *top right* panel with lateral view of distractor placeemnt. *Middle* panels - left with frontal clinical images at 1 week, right with lateral view and bottom panel, with clinical pcitures at 2 weeks postoperatively (*left panel* frontal view, *right panel* birds eye view. (*E*) CT and clinical photos of sequence—preoperative, post–strip craniectomy, and post–posterior vault distraction; post–fronto- orbital advancement. *Left* panel demonstrates preoperative state - *left top* panel is birds eye view, second is lateral view and 3rd is posterior view CT scan. *Left bottom* 4th/5th panels are oblique and frontal clinical views. FOA, fronto-orbital advancement; PVD, posterior vault distraction; VSP, virtual surgical planning.

synostoses.[85–87] Of paramount importance in early intervention for multisuture synostosis with facial dysmorphisms is the need for corneal protection and alleviating cranial constriction.[2,58,59,69,77,88] When additional sutures are involved, the common forehead retrusion, tall, shortened (turribrachycephaly) head morphology is more evident with potentially worsened asymmetry and symptoms.

For turribrachycephaly, hybrid paradigms have emerged as recommended approaches by expert experience. Early posterior vault distraction followed by interval cranial vault remodeling has been reported to lead to resolution of elevated ICP, expansion of the intracranial volume, and improved clinical outcome.[58,72,83,84,89–95] Timing of posterior vault distraction varies in the literature but is recommended at 3 months to 6 months of age with calvarial development balanced against evidence of elevated ICP.[72,84,93,94] Swanson and colleagues[93] report that approximately 40% of patients treated with this paradigm may avoid secondary cranial vault remodeling via fronto-orbital advancement given the degree of correction achieved.

CRANIAL VAULT REMODELING

Additional suture synostosis remodeling is carried out based on timing and preferred approaches, with an emphasis on complete and stable release of restricted suture by 12 months of age to allow brain growth and cranial remodeling after posterior vault distraction. Ongoing studies into developmental and neurocognitive outcomes suggest greater release and remodeling of the cranium lead to improved developmental outcomes.[42,49,50,96–98] Prior studies have demonstrated increased rates of revisionary cranioplasty in syndromic patients with this need attributed to the increased severity of the antecedent deformity.[2,84,94,99,100] Given the wide spectrum of neurocognitive presentation, lowered incidence numbers, multiple surgeries, and environmental factors that comprise any 1 syndrome, adequate long-term outcomes on the developmental influence of single suture correction for even the common syndromes. Most outcomes studies have focused on multisuture synostosis and evaluated cranial morphology, neurologic findings (papilledema and Chiari malformation), and complications associated with interventions.[41,58,72–74,78,101–105]

SURGICAL TECHNIQUES AND APPROACHES
Bicoronal Synostosis

Premature closure may occur either unilaterally or bilaterally. Bicoronal craniosynostosis is known as turribrachycephaly and is most commonly associated with syndromic craniosynostosis. The cranial deformity presents as calvarium that is shortened in the anterioposterior dimension and flattened and tall in the vertical dimension. This results from the arrest of growth in the perpendicular plane to the fused sutures. Both orbits are also affected with vertical elongation of the bones and flattened upper face.

In unicoronal synostosis, restriction of the calvarium and orbit proceed along stereotypic patterning, with flattening of the frontoparietal bone and growth restriction leading to the harlequin deformity of the orbit and deviation of the nasal root toward the affected side. Contralateral frontal and posterior bossing is often noted.

Surgical correction of coronal synostosis:

- Supine positioning
- Bicoronal incision
  - Elevation of scalp flaps in a subgaleal plane
- Elevation of laterally based pericranial flaps
  - If luckenschadel calvarial deformities are noted, extra care must be taken with subperiosteal dissection.

- Bifrontal and parietal craniotomies
  - In unilateral cases, if contralateral frontal bossing is not significant, a unilateral fronto-orbital advancement may be considered.
- Subperiosteal dissection with preservation of the supraorbital neurovascular bundle
  - May require dissection of the nerve out of the foramen
- Subperiosteal dissection of the fronto-orbital bandeau
  - Strategies for positioning/advancement include
    - Contouring of the fronto-orbital bandeau
    - Repositioning of bandeau to an over-corrected position.
    - Tilt of the fronto-orbital bandeau
- Reshaping/repositioning of the supraorbital bandeau, frontal, and parietal bones to match an improved contour
  - In unilateral coronal, correction of the flattening and harlequin deformity
  - Bicoronal synostosis requires posterior vault expansion and shortening of the vertical height of the calvarium.
  - Use of resorbable plates and suture fixation to secure the repositioned bones.

Morphometric and outcomes studies illustrate the risks and benefits of these various strategies.[50,104,106–109] Over-correction to counter expected relapse and preservation of periosteal blood supply are important considerations in achieving stable long-term results.[110]

Correction of coronal synostosis with early posterior vault distraction osteogenesis has been described, as discussed previously.[77,88] The benefit of limited calvarial bone disruption is weighed against the need for multiple surgical interventions, incremental relief of ICP, and degree of calvarial correction. Outcomes suggest improved correction and maintenance of bony correction.[111]

Early posterior vault distraction has developed into an important surgical step that allows for relief of elevated intracranial pressure and allows for improved calvarial shape. In a retrospective review of 30 patients comparing traditional fronto-orbital advancement to posterior cranial vault distraction, greater cranial vault volume was reported when adjusted for age.[77] Long-term outcomes, evaluation of facial balance, and evaluation of neurocognitive outcomes remain, however, open questions.

Posterior vault distraction:

- Prone positioning
- Bicoronal incision

- Scalp flap elevation at the level of the galea
  - May also use subperiosteal flap elevation for additional layer of coverage over distraction devices
- Subperiosteal dissection with preservation of blood supply
- Parieto-temporo-occipital bone craniotomy
- Placement of distraction devices
  - Careful analysis and placement of distraction devices in the desired vector of augmentation must be carefully considered.
- Tension-free, multilayered closure

Critical components of cranial vault restoration include

- Establishing adequate cranial height
- Correcting occipital bossing
- Establishing biparietal width

Facial Skeleton

Correction of facial dysmorphisms is a particular challenge in this patient population. Commonly performed procedures, such as Le Fort I and bilateral sagittal split osteotomies for the correction of class III maloclussion, are met with the added challenges of high arched palates, potential history of clefting, prior scarring, and high degree of asymmetry. Additional complex procedures, such as facial bipartition and box osteotomies, aim to more fully or secondarily correct hypertelorism, facial widening, and orbital malposition. These surgeries are left until the patient achieves skeletal maturity (**Table 3**).

Earlier interventions prior to skeletal maturity with distraction osteogenesis of the facial skeleton may assist in improvement of facial asymmetry; however, each intervention must be weighed against the tolerance of complex postoperative care, baseline functioning, and the psychosocial effects of multiple surgical interventions. Innovative surgical approaches aimed at correcting severe obstructive sleep apnea and facial growth restriction include monobloc advancement, Le Fort III, combined Le Fort III and Le Fort I osteotomies, Le fort III and split zygoma.[112–114] The authors' preferred approach include Le Fort III combined with Le Fort I, bilateral sagittal split osteotomy if able to fully correct the facial deformity, including occlusal discrepancies (**Fig. 4**). The monobloc advancement is an important tool; however, if a well-done fronto-orbital advancement has already taken place, this may over-correct or displace the upper third of the face and nose. A key subdivision of

Table 3
Surgical corrective options for midface dysmorphism

Midface findings	Exorbitism Exposure keratopathy OSA/airway obstruction Tracheostomy Short radix-tip Anterior cross-bite
Surgical goals	Increase volume • Reposition, advance, overcorrect midface Orbital protection Nasal and pharyngeal airway Decannulate Normalize nasal length Positive overjet
Surgical approach to midface correction	Advancement, lengthening via: • Le Fort III • Monobloc • Component surgical correction • Combination Le Fort III, Le Fort I DO

Abbreviation: DO, distraction osteogenesis.

the Le Fort III advancement is the use of differential midface advancement via the zygomas, which may allow for improved correction in cases with significant assymetry.[114]

Detailed characterization of the orbital deformity and midface hypoplasia was reported by Forte and colleagues.[115,116] These reports detail the landmark relationships that demonstrate altered sphenoid morphology; flattened, wide maxilla; and shortened orbital bones with decreased volumes that characterize the stereotypic deformities found in Apert and Crouzon. Forte and colleagues[114,115] present data from 19 patients and note the range of deformity that may be present compared with controls. Although most surgical approaches to the facial skeleton are undertaken once facial growth has stabilized, Ahmad and colleagues[117] report on outcomes after monobloc advancement in 12 patients under 3 years old for severe, functionally compromised cases.[118] Although this approach carries with it significant potential added difficulty and morbidity, it challenges current surgical convention and may yet yield an optimal solution for select cases.[71,119–123]

Importantly, secondary procedures, including cranial and facial adjuncts, are needed to set patients' occlusion and facial balance. Orthognathic surgery often marks a major milestone in the surgical journey for patients, because it is often the last 1 to 2 major procedures patients undergo, once they are skeletally mature.

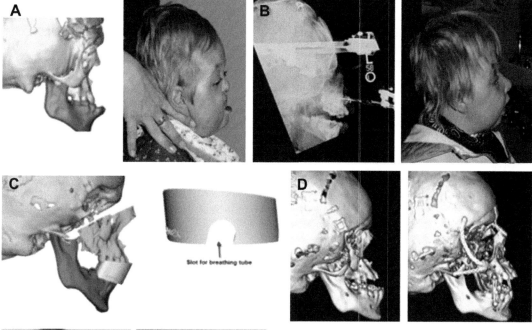

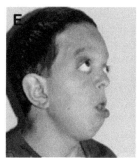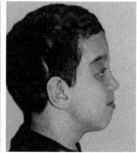

Fig. 4. Midface correction with compound Le Fort III, Le Fort I distraction osteogenesis. (*A*) Preoperative CT (*left*) and lateral photograph (*right*). (*B*) Lateral X-rya of Le Fort III distraction with RED (Rapid External Distraction) device (*left panel*) and postoperative result (*right panel*). (*C*) Use of intraoperative splint with slot for endotracheal tube (Left panel is CT of splint in place, and right sided demonstrates the splint with the slot for the endotracheal tube). (*D*) Preoperative (left) and postoperative (*right*) CT after 1-stage Le Fort III. (*E*) Preoperative (*left*) and postoperative (*right*) clinical photographs of 1-stage Le Fort III.

SUMMARY

Syndromic craniosynostosis encompasses an ever-evolving set of new genetic mutations that involve multisystem findings. In addition to premature cranial suture fusion, key characteristics include extremity findings, facial dysmorphology, potential cardiac anomalies, and neurocognitive deficiencies. Multidisciplinary team evaluation is critical in the complex care needs of these patients and assists in determining the appropriate surgical approach to complex cranial vault corrections.

REFERENCES

1. Kutkowska-Kazmierczak A, Gos M, Obersztyn E. Craniosynostosis as a clinical and diagnostic problem: molecular pathology and genetic counseling. J Appl Genet 2018;59:133–47.

2. Taylor JA, Bartlett SP. What's new in syndromic craniosynostosis surgery? Plast Reconstr Surg 2017; 140:82e–93e.

3. Cohen MM Jr. Craniosynostoses: phenotypic/molecular correlations. Am J Med Genet 1995;56:334–9.

4. Azoury SC, Reddy S, Shukla V, et al. Fibroblast growth factor receptor 2 (FGFR2) mutation related syndromic craniosynostosis. Int J Biol Sci 2017; 13:1479–88.

5. Motch Perrine SM, Stecko T, Neuberger T, et al. Integration of brain and skull in prenatal mouse models of apert and crouzon syndromes. Front Hum Neurosci 2017;11:369.

6. Maximino LP, Ducati LG, Abramides DVM, et al. Syndromic craniosynostosis: neuropsycholinguistic abilities and imaging analysis of the central nervous system. Arq Neuropsiquiatr 2017;75:862–8.

7. McKusick and Hamosh. Online Mendelian Inheritance in Man [OMIM]. Available at: http://www.omim.org. Accessed June 26, 2018.

8. Wang JC, Nagy L, Demke JC. Syndromic craniosynostosis. Facial Plast Surg Clin North Am 2016;24: 531–43.

9. Derderian C, Seaward J. Syndromic craniosynostosis. Semin Plast Surg 2012;26:64–75.

10. Gracia A, Arsuaga JL, Martínez I, et al. Craniosynostosis in the middle pleistocene human cranium 14 from the Sima de los Huesos, Atapuerca, Spain. Proc Natl Acad Sci U S A 2009;106:6573–8.

11. Pospihilova B, Prochazkova O. Paleopathological findings of dry skulls with plagiocephaly. Acta Medica (Hradec Kralove) 2006;49:219–26.

12. Gerszten PC, Gerszten E, Allison MJ. Diseases of the skull in pre-Columbian South American mummies. Neurosurgery 1998;42:1145–51 [discussion: 1151–2].

13. Bennett KA. Craniostenosis: a review of the etiology and a report of new cases. Am J Phys Anthropol 1967;27:1–10.

14. Braverman IM, Redford DB, Mackowiak PA. Akhenaten and the strange physiques of Egypt's 18th dynasty. Ann Intern Med 2009;150:556–60.

15. Di Rocco C. Craniosynostosis in old Greece: political power and physical deformity. Childs Nerv Syst 2005;21:859.

16. Lane L. Pioneer cran for relief of mental imbecility due to premature sutural closure and microcephalous. JAMA 1892;18:49–50.

17. Goodrich JT, Tutino M. An annotated history of craniofacial surgery and intentional cranial deformation. Neurosurg Clin N Am 2001;12:45–68, viii.

18. Otto A. Lehrbuch der pathologischen anatomie. Berlin: Rucher; 1830.

19. Virchow R. Ueber den Cretinismus, namentlich in Franken: und ueber pathologische Schadelformen. Verh Phys Med Gesamte Wurzburg 1851; 2:230–70.

20. Persing JA, Jane JA, Shaffrey M. Virchow and the pathogenesis of craniosynostosis: a translation of his original work. Plast Reconstr Surg 1989;83: 738–42.

21. Delashaw JB, Persing JA, Broaddus WC, et al. Cranial vault growth in craniosynostosis. J Neurosurg 1989;70:159–65.

22. Teng P. Premature synostosis of the sagittal suture, and its treatment. A modification of the linear craniectomy and the use of synthetic fabrics. J Neurosurg 1962;19:1094–7.

23. Marchac D. Radical forehead remodeling for craniostenosis. Plast Reconstr Surg 1978;61:823–35.

24. Tessier P. The definitive plastic surgical treatment of the severe facial deformities of craniofacial dysostosis. Crouzon's and Apert's diseases. Plast Reconstr Surg 1971;48:419–42.

25. Tessier P, Guiot G, Rougerie J, et al. Hypertelorism: cranio-naso-orbito-facial and subethmoid osteotomy. Panminerva Med 1969;11:102–16.

26. Tessier P, Guiot G, Derome P. Orbital hypertelorism. II. Definite treatment of orbital hypertelorism (OR.H.) by craniofacial or by extracranial osteotomies. Scand J Plast Reconstr Surg 1973;7: 39–58.

27. Tessier P. Total osteotomy of the middle third of the face for faciostenosis or for sequelae of Le Fort 3 fractures. Plast Reconstr Surg 1971;48:533–41.

28. Tessier P. The classic reprint. Experimental study of fractures of the upper jaw. I and II. Rene Le Fort, M.D. Plast Reconstr Surg 1972;50:497–506. contd.

29. Tessier P. The classic reprint: experimental study of fractures of the upper jaw. 3. Rene Le Fort, M.D., Lille, France. Plast Reconstr Surg 1972;50:600–7.

30. Tessier P. Colobomas: vertical and oblique complete facial clefts. Simultaneous operation of the eyelid, inner canthus, cheek nose and lip Orbitomaxillary bone graft. Panminerva Med 1969;11:95–101.

31. Tessier P, Tulasne JF. Stability in correction of hypertelorbitism and Treacher Collins syndromes. Clin Plast Surg 1989;16:195–204.

32. Tessier P. Inferior orbitotomy. A new approach to the orbital floor. Clin Plast Surg 1982;9:569–75.

33. Tessier P. Autogenous bone grafts taken from the calvarium for facial and cranial applications. Clin Plast Surg 1982;9:531–8.

34. Tessier P. Aesthetic aspects of bone grafting to the face. Clin Plast Surg 1981;8:279–301.

35. Tessier P, Tulasne JF, Delaire J, et al. Therapeutic aspects of maxillonasal dysostosis (Binder syndrome). Head Neck Surg 1981;3:207–15.

36. Tessier P. Compatibility between primary cranial surgery and secondary cranio-facial surgery (author's transl). Neurochirurgie 1981;27:103–13 [in French].

37. Tessier P, Tulasne JF, Delaire J, et al. Treatment of Binder's maxillonasal dysostosis (author's transl). Rev Stomatol Chir Maxillofac 1979;80:363–72 [in French].

38. Tessier P. Orbital hypertelorism. Fortschr Kiefer Gesichtschir 1974;18:14–27.

39. Tessier P. Relationship of craniostenoses to craniofacial dysostoses, and to faciostenoses: a study with therapeutic implications. Plast Reconstr Surg 1971;48:224–37.

40. Sharma VP, Fenwick AL, Brockop MS, et al. Mutations in TCF12, encoding a basic helix-loop-helix partner of TWIST1, are a frequent cause of coronal craniosynostosis. Nat Genet 2013;45:304–7.

41. Coll G, Sakka L, Botella C, et al. Pattern of closure of skull base synchondroses in crouzon syndrome. World Neurosurg 2018;109:e460–7.

42. Timberlake AT, Furey CG, Choi J, et al. De novo mutations in inhibitors of Wnt, BMP, and Ras/ERK signaling pathways in non-syndromic midline craniosynostosis. Proc Natl Acad Sci U S A 2017; 114:E7341–7.

43. Zollino M, Lattante S, Orteschi D, et al. Syndromic craniosynostosis can define new candidate genes for suture development or result from the nonspecifc effects of pleiotropic genes: rasopathies

and chromatinopathies as examples. Front Neurosci 2017;11:587.

44. Runyan CM, Xu W, Alperovich M, et al. Minor suture fusion in syndromic craniosynostosis. Plast Reconstr Surg 2017;140:434e–45e.

45. Timberlake AT, Choi J, Zaidi S, et al. Two locus inheritance of non-syndromic midline craniosynostosis via rare SMAD6 and common BMP2 alleles. Elife 2016;5. https://doi.org/10.7554/eLife.20125.

46. Pfaff MJ, Xue K, Li L, et al. FGFR2c-mediated ERK-MAPK activity regulates coronal suture development. Dev Biol 2016;415:242–50.

47. Brenig B, Schutz E, Hardt M, et al. A 20 bp duplication in Exon 2 of the aristaless-like homeobox 4 gene (ALX4) is the candidate causative mutation for tibial hemimelia syndrome in galloway cattle. PLoS One 2015;10:e0129208.

48. Clarke CM, Fok VT, Gustafson JA, et al. Single suture craniosynostosis: identification of rare variants in genes associated with syndromic forms. Am J Med Genet A 2018;176:290–300.

49. Brooks ED, Beckett JS, Yang J, et al. The etiology of neuronal development in craniosynostosis: a working hypothesis. J Craniofac Surg 2018;29: 49–55.

50. Yang JF, Brooks ED, Hashim PW, et al. The severity of deformity in metopic craniosynostosis is correlated with the degree of neurologic dysfunction. Plast Reconstr Surg 2017;139:442–7.

51. Giancotti A, D'Ambrosio V, De Filippis A, et al. Comparison of ultrasound and magnetic resonance imaging in the prenatal diagnosis of Apert syndrome: report of a case. Childs Nerv Syst 2014;30:1445–8.

52. Benn P. Expanding non-invasive prenatal testing beyond chromosomes 21, 18, 13, X and Y. Clin Genet 2016;90:477–85.

53. Benn P, Chapman AR. Ethical and practical challenges in providing noninvasive prenatal testing for chromosome abnormalities: an update. Curr Opin Obstet Gynecol 2016;28: 119–24.

54. Benn P, Curnow KJ, Chapman S, et al. An economic analysis of cell-free DNA non-invasive prenatal testing in the us general pregnancy population. PLoS One 2015;10:e0132313.

55. Gross SJ, Ryan A, Benn P. Noninvasive prenatal testing for 22q11.2 deletion syndrome: deeper sequencing increases the positive predictive value. Am J Obstet Gynecol 2015;213:254–5.

56. Benn P. Non-invasive prenatal testing using cell free DNA in maternal plasma: recent developments and future prospects. J Clin Med 2014;3:537–65.

57. Sharma RK. Craniosynostosis. Indian J Plast Surg 2013;46:18–27.

58. Ter Maaten NS, Mazzaferro DM, Wes AM, et al. A craniometric analysis of frontal cranial morphology following posterior vault distraction. J Craniofac Surg 2018. https://doi.org/10.1097/SCS.0000000000004473.

59. Mazzaferro DM, Naran S, Wes AM, et al. Incidence of cranial base suture fusion in infants with craniosynostosis. Plast Reconstr Surg 2018;141: 559e–70e.

60. Steinbacher DM. Three-dimensional analysis and surgical planning in craniomaxillofacial surgery. J Oral Maxillofac Surg 2015;73:S40–56.

61. Eley KA, Watt-Smith SR, Sheerin F, et al. "Black Bone" MRI: a potential alternative to CT with three-dimensional econstruction of the craniofacial skeleton in the diagnosis of craniosynostosis. Eur Radiol 2014;24:2417–26.

62. Kuusela L, Hukki A, Brandstack N, et al. Use of black-bone MRI in the diagnosis of the patients with posterior plagiocephaly. Childs Nerv Syst 2018. https://doi.org/10.1007/s00381-018-3783-0.

63. Suchyta MA, Gibreel W, Hunt CH, et al. Utilizing "Black Bone" MRI in craniofacial virtual surgical planning: a comparative cadaver study. Plast Reconstr Surg 2018. https://doi.org/10.1097/PRS.0000000000004396.

64. Dremmen MHG, Wagner MW, Bosemani T, et al. Does the addition of a "black bone" sequence to a fast multisequence trauma MR protocol allow MRI to replace ct after traumatic brain injury in children? AJNR Am J Neuroradiol 2017;38:2187–92.

65. Eley KA, Watt-Smith SR, Golding SJ. "Black Bone" MRI: a novel imaging technique for 3D printing. Dentomaxillofac Radiol 2017;46:20160407.

66. Eley KA, Watt-Smith SR, Golding SJ. "Black bone" MRI: a potential alternative to CT when imaging the head and neck: report of eight clinical cases and review of the Oxford experience. Br J Radiol 2012;85:1457–64.

67. Jane JA Jr, Krieger MD, Persing J. Introduction: craniosynostosis: modern treatment strategies. Neurosurg Focus 2015;38:E1.

68. Mardini S, Alsubaie S, Cayci C, et al. Three-dimensional preoperative virtual planning and template use for surgical correction of craniosynostosis. J Plast Reconstr Aesthet Surg 2014;67:336–43.

69. Derderian CA, Wink JD, Cucchiara A, et al. The temporal region in unilateral coronal craniosynostosis: a volumetric study of short- and long-term changes after fronto-orbital advancement. Plast Reconstr Surg 2014;134:83–91.

70. Beckett JS, Brooks ED, Lacadie C, et al. Altered brain connectivity in sagittal craniosynostosis. J Neurosurg Pediatr 2014;13:690–8.

71. Visser R, Ruff CF, Angullia F, et al. Evaluating the efficacy of monobloc distraction in the crouzonpfeiffer craniofacial deformity using geometric morphometrics. Plast Reconstr Surg 2017;139: 477e–87e.

72. Tomita S, Miyawaki T, Nonaka Y, et al. Surgical strategy for Apert syndrome: retrospective study of developmental quotient and three-dimensional computerized tomography. Congenit Anom (Kyoto) 2017;57:104–8.

73. McMillan K, Lloyd M, Evans M, et al. Experiences in performing posterior calvarial distraction. J Craniofac Surg 2017;28:664–9.

74. Hersh DS, Hoover-Fong JE, Beck N, et al. Endoscopic surgery for patients with syndromic craniosynostosis and the requirement for additional open surgery. J Neurosurg Pediatr 2017;20:91–8.

75. Brooks ED, Yang J, Beckett JS, et al. Normalization of brain morphology after surgery in sagittal craniosynostosis. J Neurosurg Pediatr 2016;17:460–8.

76. Zhang G, Tan H, Qian X, et al. A systematic approach to predicting spring force for sagittal craniosynostosis surgery. J Craniofac Surg 2016;27:636–43.

77. Derderian CA, Wink JD, McGrath JL, et al. Volumetric changes in cranial vault expansion: comparison of fronto-orbital advancement and posterior cranial vault distraction osteogenesis. Plast Reconstr Surg 2015;135:1665–72.

78. Satoh K, Mitsukawa N, Kubota Y, et al. Appropriate indication of fronto-orbital advancement by distraction osteogenesis in syndromic craniosynostosis: beyond the conventional technique. J Craniomaxillofac Surg 2015;43:2079–84. Elsevier Ltd.

79. van der Vlugt JJ, van der Meulen JJ, van den Braak RR, et al. Insight into the pathophysiologic mechanisms behind cognitive dysfunction in trigonocephaly. Plast Reconstr Surg 2017;139:954e–64e.

80. Dixon RR, Nocera M, Zolotor AJ, et al. Intracranial pressure monitoring in infants and young children with traumatic brain injury. Pediatr Crit Care Med 2016;17:1064–72.

81. Huang YH, Ou CY. Prognostic impact of intracranial pressure monitoring after primary decompressive craniectomy for traumatic brain injury. World Neurosurg 2016;88:59–63.

82. Mehta A, Kochanek PM, Tyler-Kabara E, et al. Relationship of intracranial pressure and cerebral perfusion pressure with outcome in young children after severe traumatic brain injury. Dev Neurosci 2010;32:413–9.

83. LoPresti M, Buchanan EP, Shah V, et al. Complete resolution of papilledema in syndromic craniosynostosis with posterior cranial vault distraction. J Pediatr Neurosci 2017;12:199–202.

84. Steinbacher DM, Skirpan J, Puchala J, et al. Expansion of the posterior cranial vault using distraction osteogenesis. Plast Reconstr Surg 2011;127:792–801.

85. Fearon JA, Griner D, Ditthakasem K, et al. Autogenous bone reconstruction of large secondary skull defects. Plast Reconstr Surg 2017;139:427–38.

86. Fearon JA. Evidence-based medicine: craniosynostosis. Plast Reconstr Surg 2014;133:1261–75.

87. Fearon JA, Podner C. Apert syndrome: evaluation of a treatment algorithm. Plast Reconstr Surg 2013;131:132–42.

88. Tahiri Y, Swanson JW, Taylor JA. Distraction osteogenesis versus conventional fronto-orbital advancement for the treatment of unilateral coronal synostosis: a comparison of perioperative morbidity and short-term outcomes. J Craniofac Surg 2015;26:1904–8.

89. Persing JA, Babler WJ, Nagorsky MJ, et al. Skull expansion in experimental craniosynostosis. Plast Reconstr Surg 1986;78:594–603.

90. David L, Glazier S, Pyle J, et al. Classification system for sagittal craniosynostosis. J Craniofac Surg 2009;20:279–82.

91. Guimaraes-Ferreira J, Gewalli F, David L, et al. Spring-mediated cranioplasty compared with the modified pi-plasty for sagittal synostosis. Scand J Plast Reconstr Surg Hand Surg 2003;37:208–15.

92. David LR, Gewalli F, Guimãraes-Ferreira J, et al. Dynamic spring-mediated cranioplasty in a rabbit model. J Craniofac Surg 2002;13:794–801.

93. Thomas GP, Wall SA, Jayamohan J, et al. Lessons learned in posterior cranial vault distraction. J Craniofac Surg 2014;25:1721–7.

94. Swanson JW, Samra F, Bauder A, et al. An algorithm for managing syndromic craniosynostosis using posterior vault distraction osteogenesis. Plast Reconstr Surg 2016;137:829e–41e.

95. Nowinski D, Saiepour D, Leikola J, et al. Posterior cranial vault expansion performed with rapid distraction and time-reduced consolidation in infants with syndromic craniosynostosis. Childs Nerv Syst 2011;27:1999–2003.

96. Xu W, Li J, Gerety PA, et al. Impact of fronto-orbital advancement on frontal sinus volume, morphology, and disease in nonsyndromic craniosynostosis. Plast Reconstr Surg 2016. https://doi.org/10.1097/PRS.0000000000002636.

97. Hashim PW, Brooks ED, Persing JA, et al. Direct brain recordings reveal impaired neural function in infants with single-suture craniosynostosis: a future modality for guiding management? J Craniofac Surg 2015;26:60–3.

98. Patel A, Yang JF, Hashim PW, et al. The impact of age at surgery on long-term neuropsychological outcomes in sagittal craniosynostosis. Plast Reconstr Surg 2014;134:608e–17e.

99. Goldstein JA, Paliga JT, Taylor JA, et al. Complications in 54 frontofacial distraction procedures in patients with syndromic craniosynostosis. J Craniofac Surg 2015;26:124–8.

100. Whitaker LA, Bartlett SP. The craniofacial dysostoses: guidelines for management of the symmetric and asymmetric deformities. Clin Plast Surg 1987; 14:73–81.

101. Morrison KA, Lee JC, Souweidane MM, et al. Twenty-year outcome experience with open craniosynostosis repairs: an analysis of reoperation and complication rates. Ann Plast Surg 2018;80: S158–63.

102. Abraham P, Brandel MG, Dalle Ore CL, et al. Predictors of postoperative complications of craniosynostosis repair in the national inpatient sample. Ann Plast Surg 2018;80:S261–6.

103. Prada-Madrid JR, Franco-Chaparro LP, Garcia-Wenninger M, et al. A Surgical technique for management of the metopic suture in syndromic craniosynostosis. J Craniofac Surg 2017;28: 675–8.

104. Patel KB, Skolnick GB, Mulliken JB. Anthropometric outcomes following fronto-orbital advancement for metopic synostosis. Plast Reconstr Surg 2016; 137:1539–47.

105. Fearon JA, Dimas V, Ditthakasem K. Lambdoid craniosynostosis: the relationship with chiari deformations and an analysis of surgical outcomes. Plast Reconstr Surg 2016;137:946–51.

106. Yee ST, Fearon JA, Gosain AK, et al. Classification and management of metopic craniosynostosis. J Craniofac Surg 2015;26:1812–7.

107. Ezaldein HH, Metzler P, Persing JA, et al. Three-dimensional orbital dysmorphology in metopic synostosis. J Plast Reconstr Aesthet Surg 2014;67: 900–5.

108. Patel A, Chang CC, Terner JS, et al. Improved correction of supraorbital rim deformity in craniosynostosis by the "tilt" procedure. J Craniofac Surg 2012;23:370–3.

109. Czerwinski M, Kolar JC, Fearon JA. Complex craniosynostosis. Plast Reconstr Surg 2011;128: 955–61.

110. Metzler P, Ezaldein HH, Persing JA, et al. Comparing two fronto-orbital advancement strategies to treat trigonocephaly in metopic synostosis. J Craniomaxillofac Surg 2014;42:1437–41. Elsevier Ltd.

111. Jeong WS, Choi JW, Oh TS, et al. Long-term follow-up of one-piece fronto-orbital advancement with distraction but without a bandeau for coronal craniosynostosis: Review of 26 consecutive cases. J Craniomaxillofac Surg 2016;44(9):1252–8.

112. Forrest CR, Hopper RA. Craniofacial syndromes and surgery. Plast Reconstr Surg 2013;131: 86e–109e.

113. Hopper RA. New trends in cranio-orbital and midface distraction for craniofacial dysostosis. Curr Opin Otolaryngol Head Neck Surg 2012;20: 298–303.

114. Hopper RA, Prucz RB, Iamphongsai S. Achieving differential facial changes with Le Fort III distraction osteogenesis: the use of nasal passenger grafts, cerclage hinges, and segmental movements. Plast Reconstr Surg 2012;130:1281–8.

115. Forte AJ, Steinbacher DM, Persing JA, et al. Orbital dysmorphology in untreated children with crouzon and apert syndromes. Plast Reconstr Surg 2015; 136:1054–62.

116. Forte AJ, Alonso N, Persing JA, et al. Analysis of midface retrusion in Crouzon and Apert syndromes. Plast Reconstr Surg 2014;134:285–93.

117. Ahmad F, Cobb AR, Mills C, et al. Frontofacial monobloc distraction in the very young: a review of 12 consecutive cases. Plast Reconstr Surg 2012;129:488e–97e.

118. Glass GE, Ruff CF, Crombag GAJC, et al. The role of bipartition distraction in the treatment of apert syndrome. Plast Reconstr Surg 2018;141:747–50.

119. Khonsari RH, Way B, Nysjö J, et al. Fronto-facial advancement and bipartition in Crouzon-Pfeiffer and Apert syndromes: impact of fronto-facial surgery upon orbital and airway parameters in FGFR2 syndromes. J Craniomaxillofac Surg 2016; 44:1567–75.

120. Gwanmesia I, Jeelani O, Hayward R, et al. Fronto-facial advancement by distraction osteogenesis: a long-term review. Plast Reconstr Surg 2015;135: 553–60.

121. Britto JA, Greig A, Abela C, et al. Frontofacial surgery in children and adolescents: techniques, indications, outcomes. Semin Plast Surg 2014;28: 121–9.

122. Cobb AR, Boavida P, Docherty R, et al. Monobloc and bipartition in craniofacial surgery. J Craniofac Surg 2013;24:242–6.

123. Dunaway DJ, Britto JA, Abela C, et al. Complications of frontofacial advancement. Childs Nerv Syst 2012;28:1571–6.

Orthognathic Surgery for Patients with Cleft Lip and Palate

Andree-Anne Roy, MD, MSc, FRCSC[a],
Michael Alexander Rtshiladze, BSc(Med), MBBS, MS, FRACS[b],
Kyle Stevens, BSc, DDS, MSc, FRCDC[c],
John Phillips, BSc, MA, MD, FRCSC[d],*

KEYWORDS

• Orthognathic • Orthodontic • Cleft • Lip • Cleft palate • Alveolar bone graft • Distraction • Fistula

KEY POINTS

- Cleft patients present with common anatomic differences, such as a maxilla deficiency in all 3 axes, that arise from intrinsic factors and as a result of previous surgery.
- Alveolar bone grafting is an important procedure in the treatment plan of a cleft patient, and its successful completion will have great influence on later orthognathic surgery.
- Careful orthodontic planning involves devising strategies to deal with cleft dental differences, residual oronasal fistulae, and alveolar segment incoordination.
- When dealing with cleft patients, surgical technique must be altered in terms of the planned incision, provision for fistula repair, and approach to dealing with soft tissue restriction, limiting advancement.
- Complications from orthognathic surgery in a cleft population are similar to those in the general population, with an increased risk of relapse and velopharyngeal insufficiency.

INTRODUCTION

A combined orthodontic and orthognathic treatment plan is a powerful tool that can correct significant malocclusion and produce major improvements in facial aesthetics and balance. The principles and technical details of orthognathic surgery have been well described. Cleft lip and/or palate (CL/P) patients represent a unique group, with commonalities in their presentation and unique challenges in their orthognathic treatment.

This article seeks to examine some of the specific difficulties faced when treating this group and describes the differences in planning, surgery, and postoperative management encountered in this particular patient cohort.

BACKGROUND
Anatomic Characteristics

The facial skeletons of patients with CL/P possess common and characteristic findings. Cleft patients

Disclosure: The authors have no conflicts to disclose. The present study conformed to the Declaration of Helsinki.
[a] Department of Plastic and Reconstructive Surgery, Hospital for Sick Children, 555 University Avenue, Toronto, Ontario M5G 1X8, Canada; [b] Craniofacial Unit, Department of Plastic and Reconstructive Surgery, Sydney Children's Hospital, Randwick, High Street, Sydney, New South Wales 2031, Australia; [c] Orthodontics, Department of Dentistry, Hospital for Sick Children, 555 University Avenue, Toronto, Ontario M5G 1X8, Canada; [d] Division of Plastic and Reconstructive Surgery, University of Toronto, Hospital for Sick Children, 555 University Avenue, Toronto, Ontario M5G 1X8, Canada
* Corresponding author.
E-mail address: john.phillips@sickkids.ca

present with a maxilla that is deficient in all 3 dimensions and is often accompanied by constriction of the maxillary dental arch.[1] The cause of the maxillary growth disturbance is thought to be both the original intrinsic embryologic tissue defect and a result of previous surgeries.[2–4] However, it has been observed that unrepaired CL/P patients have normal maxillary growth.[5] Some investigators believe that the sole cause of hypoplasia is the multiple surgical interventions at a young age leads to subsequent scar formation and contracture.[6–8]

The severity of maxillary hypoplasia is related to cleft type.[5] In unilateral cases, the maxillary lesser segment is most commonly hypoplastic and is displaced superiorly, posteriorly, and medially. The maxillary midline is commonly deviated toward the side of the cleft. Bilateral cleft cases tend to present with an extremely narrow maxilla that results from the posterior alveolar segments collapsing medially. This can be seen clinically as a bilateral posterior cross-bite. The premaxilla may be either superiorly or inferiorly positioned and is often protruded. A differing presentation is when there is a palatally displaced premaxilla.[9] At the time of orthognathic surgery, patients with bilateral CL/P have multiple residual problems, such as scarring, agenesis of lateral incisors, alveolar defects, abnormal nasal anatomy, and upper lip muscular dysfunction.[10]

The mandibular growth is unaffected in CL/P patients. However, there is a common presentation with an anterior open bite and a steep mandibular plane angle. This is caused by a decreased posterior facial height and results in the appearance of a long anterior face.[9]

Incidence

CL/P is the most common congenital facial difference. The incidence of the need for orthognathic surgery among these patients is highly variable depending on institution and investigator. The literature demonstrates that anywhere from 14% to 75% of cleft patients undergo orthognathic surgery.[5,11–15] When considered by cleft type, the rates of orthognathic surgery are also disparate. The rate of orthognathic surgery in unilateral cleft patients is often quoted as 25%.[9] More recent publications have put the rate significantly higher with 48.3% of unilateral cleft patients undergoing orthognathic surgery in one center.[13] In that same center, 65% of patients with a repaired bilateral CL/P underwent orthognathic surgery.[13] In the isolated cleft palate population, the need for orthognathic surgery is considerably less. The reported rate of orthognathic surgery in patients with nonsyndromic isolated cleft palate is 12.5%.[16]

PREORTHOGNATHIC CONSIDERATIONS
Alveolar Bone Grafting

Alveolar bone grafting (ABG) is an important procedure in the overall treatment of CL/P patients, and its successful completion will have great influence on later orthognathic surgery. Repair of the alveolar cleft begins at mid to late mixed dentition. Midface growth restriction has been associated with primary ABG at the time of lip repair[17–19]; however, bone grafting performed at time of mixed dentition has shown no measurable impact on midface growth in several studies.[20,21] An ABG allows greater orthodontic control of alveolar segments, improves dental positioning within the maxillary arch, facilitates eruption of the cleft dentition, and closes alveolar and oronasal fistulae.[22] These effects facilitate orthodontic space closure,[23] thus simplifying future orthognathic procedures (Fig. 1). Furthermore, in appropriate patients, a successful ABG can produce a dental arch with adequate bone stock to support an osseointegrated dental implant.[24]

Before an ABG, orthodontics can be used to optimize the positions of the maxillary segments. Expansion of the maxilla is performed with the use of fixed orthodontic appliances and expanders.

In a bilateral CL/P patient with a severely displaced premaxilla, surgical repositioning may be considered in conjunction with the ABG.[11,12] Bilateral ABG with surgical premaxillary repositioning is indicated in extreme protrusion of the premaxilla, extreme vertical overdevelopment of the premaxilla, severe lateral displacement of the premaxilla, and closure of large oronasal fistula.[11] It is associated with risk of avascular necrosis, underlining the importance of minimal periosteal elevation on the premaxillary segment.

Preorthognathic Orthodontics

Combined orthodontic-orthognathic treatment requires careful planning and a multidisciplinary collaborative approach in order to achieve successful outcomes. Presurgical orthodontic treatment with preoperative decompensation[25] and postoperative refinement[26] is essential.[4]

Timing and goals of presurgical orthodontics
Orthodontic treatment can start 3 to 6 months following ABG or be planned to be completed at skeletal maturity in time for orthognathic surgery. The purpose of the presurgical orthodontic preparation is to align the dentition and remove dental

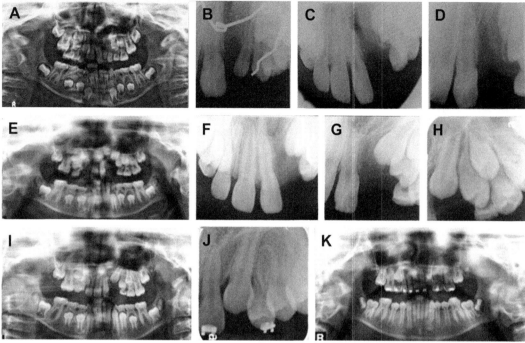

Fig. 1. Sequence of orthodontic treatment combined with ABG in a patient with unilateral CL/P. (*A*) Preexpansion panoramic radiograph. (*B*) Postexpansion periapical radiograph. (*C*) Pre-ABG occlusal radiograph. (*D*) Pre-ABG periapical radiograph. (*E*) Pre-ABG panoramic radiograph. (*F*) Five months post-ABG occlusal radiograph. (*G*) Five months post-ABG periapical radiograph. (*H*) Ten months post-ABG periapical radiograph. (*I*) Ten months post-ABG panoramic radiograph. (*J*) Initiation of orthodontic upper alignment and crowding correction periapical radiograph. (*K*) Initiation of orthodontic upper alignment and crowding correction panoramic radiograph.

compensations to attempt to achieve maximum intercuspation of the dental arches after orthognathic surgery, which supports stability.[9,27]

When orthodontic care is planned to commence following ABG, a postoperative radiograph should be performed to evaluate the quality of the bone stock surrounding the cleft adjacent teeth.[28] Uprighting of the distally tipped central incisor and mesially tipped canine should be performed with caution depending on the quality of the ABG.[29]

Orthodontic planning

Orthodontic treatment in CL/P patients must compensate for 3 commonly encountered problems: agenesis of lateral incisors, residual alveolar clefts, and a deficient maxilla.[23] The common presentation of agenesis of the cleft side lateral incisor can be dealt with in 2 ways. A decision must be made during orthodontic planning if the space is to be maintained for a dental prosthesis (such as a dental implant with crown, or bridge) or if the canine is to be moved to substitute for the missing incisor. This decision must take into consideration the occlusal relationships, the suitability of the bone stock in the alveolar ridge for accepting an osseointegrated implant, the size and shape of the canine, the state of the periodontal tissues of the cleft adjacent teeth, and the presence of oronasal fistulae.[9] Canine substitution is often a superior alternative to the compromised lateral incisors because of the better bone support, larger root structure, and improved aesthetics.[23]

One-piece Le Fort I osteotomies can be considered in cases whereby there is good alveolar continuity following previously successful ABG (**Fig. 2**). This is often possible even in bilateral cleft cases. When there is failure of the original ABG or where an ABG has not been performed, a segmental advancement surgery is often favored.[30] When patients are prepared orthodontically for segmental advancement surgery, the teeth approximating the cleft should be upright with good supporting bone on all aspects of the root surface. In patients in whom the lesser segment is to be advanced to close the cleft, it is better to upright and align the teeth, using segmental mechanics without expansion, and correct the buccal lingual incoordination surgically. Occasionally, extraction of a premolar is required to provide the proper bone support for the canine.[30]

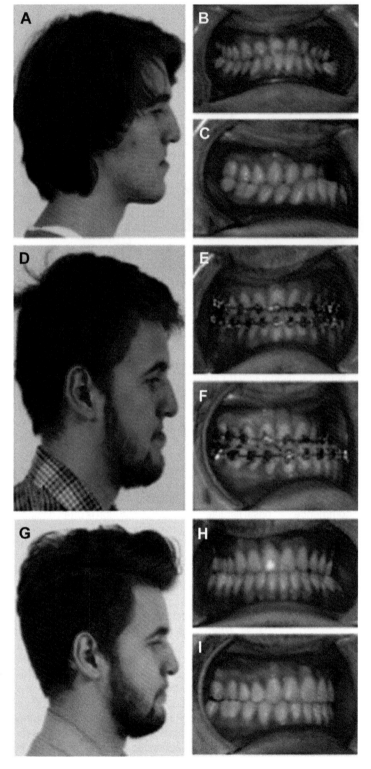

Fig. 2. Patient with unilateral CL/P had a Le Fort I one-piece 14-mm advancement osteotomy with BSSO for class III malocclusion and midline rotation. (*A*) Lateral view of CL/P patient with class III malocclusion. (*B*) Intraoral frontal view in occlusion. (*C*) Intraoral right buccal view in occlusion. (*D*) Lateral view of CL/P patient after orthodontic decompensation and alignment. (*E*) Intraoral frontal view in occlusion. (*F*) Intraoral right buccal view in occlusion. (*G*) Lateral view of CL/P patient post–Le Fort I and BSSO. (*H*) Intraoral frontal view in occlusion. (*I*) Intraoral right buccal view in occlusion.

Consideration needs to be given to each patient's dimensions in terms of sagittal, transverse, and vertical measurements. Rotational maxillary advancements may cause posterior cross-bites or arch incoordination. An asymmetric extraction may be required as part of the combined orthodontic/orthognathic treatment plan to reduce the amount of required rotation. This is particularly helpful in cases of dental crowding. When dental crowding is present in the greater segment (in unilateral cases), extraction of one premolar or lateral incisor from the noncleft segment can be considered. This may help achieve good aesthetic outcomes when there is also agenesis of the cleft side lateral incisor. Further dental extractions in this fashion can reduce the magnitude of the skeletal movement required to achieve a functional occlusion.[9]

If the surgical plan will involve segmentalizing the maxilla and closing the edentulous space, then orthodontic preparation should include uprighting of the cleft adjacent teeth. If this is not performed and the teeth are tipped severely into the cleft, then early interdental contact will occur intraoperatively. This in turn can prevent adequate bony approximation of the lesser and greater palatal segments.[31,32]

A presurgical orthodontic treatment plan should also include referral for impacted third molar removal when required.

Oral hygiene

Another important consideration with orthodontic treatment is preventive dental care. CL/P patients can exhibit poor oral hygiene. There is often enamel hypoplasia present that places these patients at an increased risk of caries.[33,34] The presence of orthodontic appliances also makes maintaining oral hygiene more difficult for patients. Cleft patients are at a greater risk of periodontal disease and often display loss of periodontal attachment. This is particularly problematic in cleft adjacent teeth, where loss of periodontal support can manifest as pathologic loosening.[35]

Preorthognathic Speech Pathology

Speech pathology assessment is an important part of the presurgical workup. This entails a clinical examination with the possible addition of nasoendoscopic study to evaluate the risk of velopharyngeal insufficiency following surgery.[8]

ORTHOGNATHIC SURGERY
Surgical Planning

The general treatment principles for cleft orthognathics are very similar to those used when performing surgery in noncleft patients. An ideal preparation involves adequate planning with cephalometric analysis, models, and an occlusal splint to allow for good postoperative occlusion in one stage after orthognathic surgery.[27,31,36]

Orthognathic surgery in the cleft patient mainly involves maxillary advancement with possible mandibular setback. The need for maxillary advancement is due to the midface deficiency that is associated with adult cleft patients. A mandibular movement is planned in several situations, namely, if the sagittal discrepancy is too great, if there is canting of the mandibular occlusal plane, or if there is significant mandibular asymmetries. Bimaxillary surgery will reduce the magnitude of both the maxillary and the mandibular movements needed to correct the underlying skeletal imbalance. This requires the fabrication of a surgical intermediate splint, for the relation of the new maxilla position to the existing mandible, and a final surgical splint, which relates the final mandibular position to the fixed final maxillary position.[31,37]

A segmental maxillary advancement can be planned during Le Fort I surgery to close the cleft. It can also be used to expand the maxillary arch posteriorly while allowing for transverse arch coordination, maximizing intercuspation and improving postoperative stability. This approach may also make the soft tissue closure of any oronasal fistulae easier by bringing the bony edges closer together and removing tension from the soft tissue repair.[22]

Surgical planning needs to consider dental anomalies often encountered in the cleft patient population. Dental changes can include variation in shape, position, and number of teeth, the presence of supernumerary teeth, and ectopic eruption of teeth.[38,39] The most frequent anomalies are agenesis of the lateral incisor and ectopic eruption of the maxillary first molars. These dental differences must be considered and accounted for when planning the final occlusion.

Dealing with the premaxilla

Bilateral CL/P patients with a palatally displaced premaxilla represent a significant technical challenge. Anterior repositioning of the premaxilla in these cases leads to an increase in the size of any oronasal fistulae and makes management of the soft tissue extremely difficult.[9] When possible, it is best to avoid this scenario by performing consolidation of the premaxilla with the lateral segments during the ABG at an earlier age.

Orthognathic Surgery Technique

Incisions

The surgical approach in a noncleft Le Fort I procedure involves an upper buccal sulcus incision. In standard cleft orthognathic cases, this incision is planned to extend vertically along the fistula margin if present. This approach is usually adequate in unilateral cleft orthognathic cases whereby the alveolar defect is narrow. In unilateral cleft cases whereby there is a significant alveolar

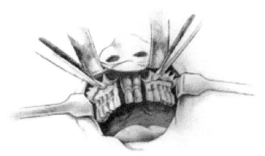

Fig. 3. Completed elevation of bilateral buccal-gingival flaps in a patient with bilateral CL/P who is undergoing a Le Fort I 3-piece osteotomy. (*From* Le-shem D, Tompson B, Phillips JH. Segmental Le Fort I surgery: turning a predicted soft-tissue failure into a success. Plast Reconstr Surg 2006;118:1213–6; with permission.)

defect, the incision can be planned similar to the approach used most often in an ABG. This is done with the elevation of a lesser segment buccal-gingival flap. A back cut and/or periosteal scoring can be performed to allow further mobilization of the soft tissues to allow for tension-free closure of the alveolus. This maneuver will usually allow for flap advancement of up to one papilla toward the cleft defect. After elevation of this flap, there is good surgical exposure to perform the Le Fort I osteotomy in the standard fashion. The use of these large mucoperiosteal flaps has been

shown to be reliable in the repair of alveolar cleft defects.[40]

In bilateral cleft cases, the initial incision is made bilaterally with preservation of the mucosa in the midline over the premaxilla (**Figs. 3** and **4**). This initially preserves an additional blood supply to the premaxilla. This incision can be extended in the standard fashion if the premaxilla is found to have bony union to the remainder of the maxilla and has a reliable vascularity.[31,32]

Osteotomies

Le Fort I advancement In cleft orthognathics, the Le Fort I osteotomy is performed in the standard fashion. A bone saw is used to perform the osteotomies of the lateral maxillary buttress and anterior wall of maxilla. The lateral nasal wall osteotomy is completed with an osteotome. The endpoint for this osteotomy is the audible change in tone when tapping with the mallet as the tip of the osteotome enters the thickened maxillary bone immediately anterior to the sphenopalatine foramen. A pterygo-maxillary disjunction is performed with a semicurved osteotome. Downfracture of the maxilla is completed with firm but constant digital pressure applied with the alveolar arch grasped bilaterally between index finger and thumb. Rowes forceps may also be used to gain additional mechanical advantage for downfracture. Following downfracture, an inspection is made of the site

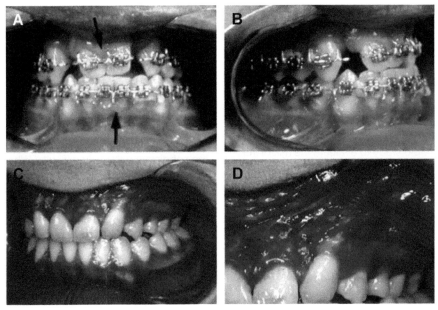

Fig. 4. Patient with bilateral CL/P had a Le Fort I 3-piece osteotomy and bilateral buccal-gingival flaps. (*A*) Intraoral frontal view in occlusion with misalignment and edentulous spaces after orthodontic decompensation. (*B*) Intraoral right buccal view in occlusion. (*C*) Intraoral left buccal view in occlusion post–Le Fort I osteotomy with bilateral buccal-gingival flaps. (*D*) Intraoral left buccal view close-up of buccal-gingival closure. *Arrows* indicate dental midline misalignment.

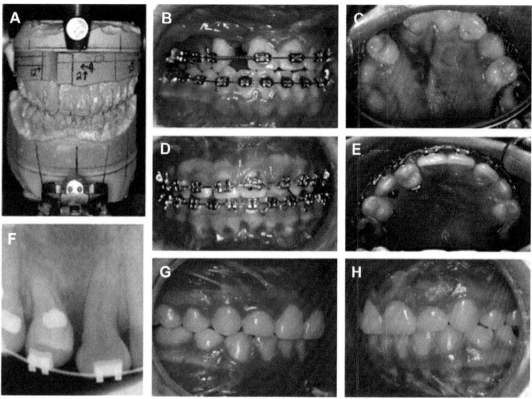

Fig. 5. Patient with unilateral CL/P had a Le Fort I 2-piece advancement osteotomy with fistula closure for class III malocclusion. (*A*) Frontal view of surgical model. (*B*) Intraoral right buccal view in occlusion with edentulous space. (*C*) Intraoral maxillary occlusal view with naso-oral fistula. (*D*) Intraoral frontal view in occlusion post–Le Fort I 2-piece advancement osteotomy with fistula closure. (*E*) Intraoral maxillary occlusal view with closed fistula. (*F*) Periapical radiograph after surgical closure of cleft and edentulous space. (*G*) Intraoral right buccal view following postsurgical orthodontics. (*H*) Intraoral left buccal view following postsurgical orthodontics.

of the fracture through the posterior maxillary wall. Any residual soft tissue attachments are freed at this time. Often the descending palatine vascular pedicle will be visible in the depth of the surgical field. In cleft orthognathic cases, a significant amount of soft tissue scarring is usually encountered. This most frequently manifests as a soft tissue restriction that minimizes the mobility of the osteotomized maxilla. The application of constant and firm traction to the soft tissues limiting the maxillary advancement for a prolonged time is essential in order to achieve adequate advancement in many cleft cases. It is imperative that the final maxillary advancement can be reached passively. First, a prefabricated interdental splint is wired to the mandibular teeth and then the mobile maxilla is set into the splint. During this maneuver, care must be taken to ensure the mandibular condyles are firmly and definitely seated in the glenoid fossae. The maxilla is temporarily wired into the splint, while rigid fixation is applied to medial and lateral buttresses. In cases

with more than 10 mm of advancement, soft tissue traction for 20 to 30 minutes may be required to ensure a passive seating of the maxilla into the interdental splint.[9] Mobilization and advancement are more difficult in bilateral CL/P cases. With large advancements, attention must be paid to the vascularity of the premaxilla.[41]

When required, segmentalization of the maxilla is performed following the Le Fort I osteotomy and downfracture. With inferiorly oriented traction on the mobile maxilla, the palatal side can be accessed. Round burs can be used to divide the maxilla along a paramedian axis. Burring of the cleft adjacent bone is often required to allow for closure of the edentulous space and adequate fit into the prepared orthodontic splint. A 2-piece (for unilateral cases) (**Figs. 5** and **6**) or a 3-piece (for bilateral cases) (**Fig. 7**) maxillary osteotomy can be created. Segmentalization of the maxilla is often accompanied by iliac crest bone grafting; especially between the lateral segments in the case of 3-piece Le Fort I to ensure for stability of

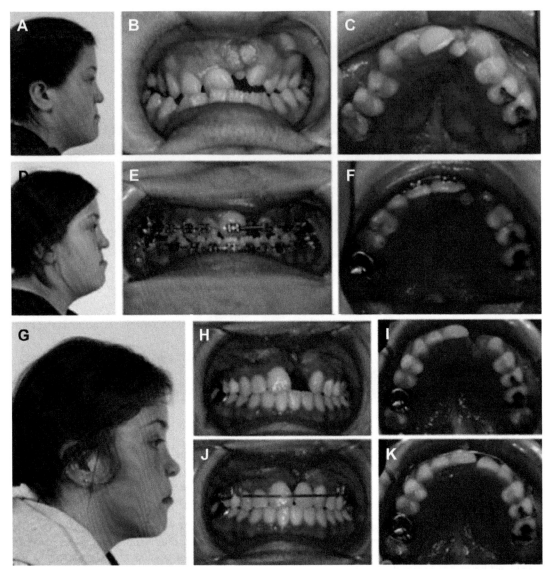

Fig. 6. Patient with unilateral CL/P had a Le Fort I 2-piece advancement osteotomy with prosthodontics for class III malocclusion. (*A*) Lateral view of CL/P patient with class III malocclusion. (*B*) Intraoral frontal view in occlusion with misalignment and crowding. (*C*) Intraoral maxillary occlusal view. (*D*) Lateral view of CL/P patient after orthodontic decompensation, extraction, and alignment. (*E*) Intraoral frontal view in occlusion. (*F*) Intraoral maxillary occlusal view. (*G*) Lateral view of CL/P patient post–Le Fort I 2-piece advancement. (*H*) Intraoral frontal view in occlusion. (*I*) Intraoral maxillary occlusal view. (*J*) Intraoral frontal view in occlusion with temporary orthodontic retainer with pontic. (*K*) Intraoral maxillary occlusal view (once stability was achieved, patient was set up with prosthodontic bridge).

the incised premaxillary segment, which has been stabilized by the surgical splint.[31,32] When there is impaction of the maxilla planned, it is not necessary to remove the entirety of the specified maxillary bone. In these cases, an attempt is made to deal with the interference by only removing the portion of lateral maxilla that is posterior to the cut edge of the superior maxilla and zygoma with the dental arch in its advanced position. In this way, the impacted and advanced maxillary arch is "locked" in front of a solid segment of bone superior to the osteotomy (**Fig. 8**).[9]

Bilateral sagittal split osteotomy Several different osteotomies have been described for the mandibular sagittal split. An effective option involves a relatively straight line cut from medial to lateral cortex. A straight line cut may reduce stress risers

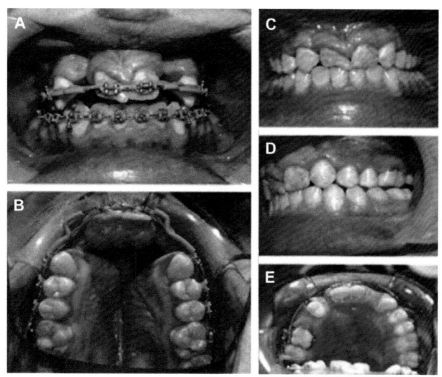

Figs. 7. (*A*) Preoperative intraoral frontal view in occlusion. (*B*) Preoperative intraoral maxillary occlusal view with a large fistula. (*C*) Postoperative intraoral frontal view in occlusion with good gingival closure. (*D*) Intraoral left buccal view in occlusion with good gingival closure with advancement. Preoperative and postoperative views of a bilateral CL/P patient for whom Le Fort I 3-piece osteotomy was planned of both lesser segments of Le Fort. (*E*) Postoperative intraoral maxillary occlusal view with closure of palatal fistula. (*From* Phillips JH, Nish I, Daskalogiannakis J. Orthognathic surgery in cleft patients. Plast Reconstr Surg 2012;129(3):542e; with permission.)

that can be induced in a more traditional stepped cut approach, and doing so may increase the risk of a favorable split (**Fig. 9**).[9] A reciprocating saw or piezoelectric device can be used to start the osteotomy. It can then be completed with a selection of fine osteotomes.

Closure of oronasal fistulae For patients with unilateral and bilateral CL/P, approximation of the maxillary segments for closure of the edentulous spaces also closed the dead space of the cleft alveolus and approximated the labial and palatal flaps to allow for straightforward closure of recalcitrant oronasal fistula without tension, while providing keratinized mucosa to surround the cleft site(s) and adjacent teeth (**Fig. 10**).[42]

Bone grafting The need for autogenous bone grafting is assessed on table following the maxillary advancement. Simultaneous corticocancellous iliac bone grafting is used to fill all residual palatal or floor of nose defects, and additional grafts are wedged between the proximal and distal parts of the zygomaticomaxillary buttresses.[42]

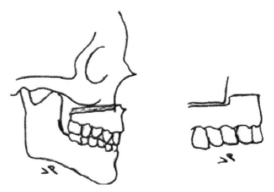

Fig. 8. When performing a Le Fort I osteotomy with advancement and impaction, all of the bone should not be removed. Only the impacted bone that is impinging and preventing the desired impaction should be removed. The bone anterior to the impingement should be left to allow locking off of the advanced segment. This still allows for removal of the impinging bone posterior to the advancement to allow for the desired impaction. (*From* Phillips JH, Nish I, Daskalogiannakis J. Orthognathic surgery in cleft patients. Plast Reconstr Surg 2012;129(3):543e; with permission.)

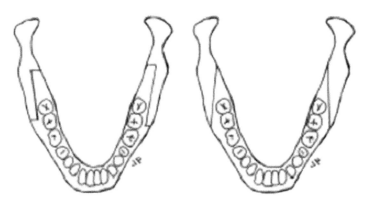

Fig. 9. (*left*) Traditional drawing of bilateral sagittal split cuts. The 90° cuts increase the stress riser in directions that could lead to a bad split. (*right*) During a BSSO, a straight-line cut is made from the medial to lateral cortex. (*From* Phillips JH, Nish I, Daskalogiannakis J. Orthognathic surgery in cleft patients. Plast Reconstr Surg 2012;129(3):543e; with permission.)

POSTOPERATIVE CONSIDERATIONS
Postsurgical Orthodontics

The interdental splint is a useful aid during the postoperative period. It can be left wired to the maxillary teeth and retained for 6 to 8 weeks postoperatively. The occlusion is not required to be held in intermaxillary fixation (IMF) because skeletal stability following Le Fort I advancement is not dependent on postoperative IMF even in CL/P patients.[41]

At the time of splint removal, the sectional arch bar can be replaced with a continuous arch wire. Brackets on the cleft adjacent teeth may also be replaced to remove compensations and begin to idealize root parallelism. Postoperative orthodontics is usually maintained for a period of 6 to 12 months. Coordinated dental arches with good intercuspation and positive overbite and overjet are important in providing skeletal stability and resisting relapse.[9]

Speech Pathology Follow-Up

Post-surgical speech pathology assessment is completed after removal of occlusal splint in the patient with increased preoperative risk of velopharyngeal insufficiency.

COMPLICATIONS

Complications from orthognathic surgery in cleft patients range from malocclusion, inferior alveolar nerve damage, inadequate or incomplete splits in bilateral sagittal split osteotomy (BSSO), postoperative bleed, velopharyngeal incompetence, and postsurgical relapse. Rare complications include blindness and stroke from Le Fort I downfracture.[31,37,43]

Relapse

Relapse following orthognathic surgery is more common among cleft patients. Relapse rate in noncleft patients with Le Fort I advancement is known to be 10%.[44] However, relapse rates in CP patients and bilateral CL/P patients have been shown to be similar.[41] After maxillary advancement by Le Fort 1 osteotomy and miniplate fixation in patients with CL/P, a certain tendency to relapse was found in about 20% to 25% 1 year after surgical correction compared with 10% in noncleft patients.[4]

Problems with long-term stability of maxillary advancement Le Fort 1 in patients with CL/P have been attributed to retraction of the scar tissue, tightness of the upper lip, interference with the nasal septum, inadequate mobilization of the bony segment, and thin and fragile bony structures of the lateral piriform wall and zygoma base for rigid fixation.[45,46] This may be the product of previous surgery, methods of fixation, neuromuscular adaptation, and orthodontics.[41] It is generally accepted that relapse tendencies start immediately after surgery up to about 6 months postoperatively. After 1 year, results can be considered stable.[4,26,47–50]

There is no significant difference in skeletal relapse in traditional cleft orthognathic surgery in single and segmental advancements.[22] Sagittal relapse following Le Fort I maxillary advancement in non-syndromic unilateral CL/P patients is independent of the amount of advancement. Relapses were not significant, because postoperative orthodontic treatment was able to compensate for the skeletal changes.[51]

Velopharyngeal Insufficiency

Patients with perceived hypernasal speech preoperatively will have hypernasal speech postoperatively. The incidence of patients with normal speech who develop velopharyngeal insufficiency postoperatively is 12.5%.[8] Preoperative hypernasality and borderline velopharyngeal insufficiency are risk factors for deterioration in function after surgery.[52,53]

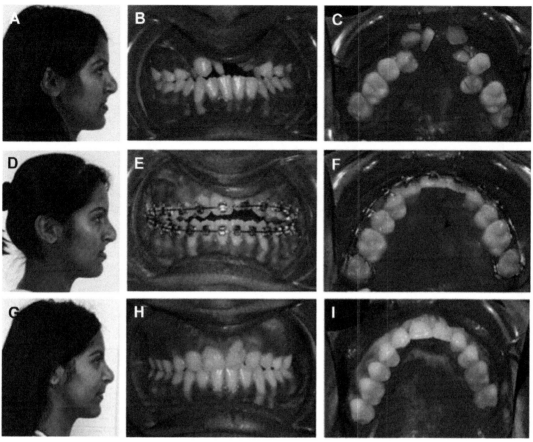

Fig. 10. Patient with bilateral CL/P and prior ABG had a Le Fort I one-piece advancement osteotomy with iliac crest bone graft and fistula closure for class III malocclusion. (*A*) Lateral view of CL/P patient with class III malocclusion. (*B*) Intraoral frontal view in occlusion with misalignment and crowding. (*C*) Intraoral maxillary occlusal view. (*D*) Lateral view of CL/P patient after orthodontic decompensation and alignment. (*E*) Intraoral frontal view in occlusion. (*F*) Intraoral maxillary occlusal view with presence of fistula. (*G*) Lateral view of CL/P patient post–Le Fort I one-piece advancement with fistula closure. (*H*) Intraoral frontal view in occlusion. (*I*) Intraoral maxillary occlusal view with closed fistula.

OTHER OPTIONS
Distraction Osteogenesis

Several surgical difficulties are encountered when applying a conventional orthognathic approach to a CL/P population. These challenges are related to the severity of scarring from previous surgeries, the less predictable vascular supply, the extent of maxillary advancement often required for these patients, and the increased risk of surgical relapse.[46] The use of osteodistraction in orthognathic surgery began in an attempt to address many of the above concerns.[4,54–58] Distraction techniques involve a gradual stretching of the soft tissues over a period of days to weeks (**Fig. 11**). Distraction can be used in cleft orthognathics to advance; a previously bone-grafted one-piece maxilla, a segmentalized maxilla, or a dentoalveolar segment. Numerous designs of both internal and external distractor devices for use in orthognathic surgery exist.[55,59] Distraction is best performed in close association with an experienced orthodontic team. The role of the orthodontist can include assistance with preoperative planning, fabrication of tooth borne retention hardware, and postoperative monitoring and vector modification.

Postoperative osteodistraction protocols commonly involve a latency period of 3 to 7 days and an activation phase with a rate of 1 mm per day in 2 to 4 rhythms. An overcorrection of at least 20% is recommended for the growing CL/P patient to compensate for relapse, residual maxillary growth deficit, and future mandibular growth.[60] A consolidation period of 2 to 3 months is common to ensure that the distraction segments heal before distractors are removed. Elastics are also

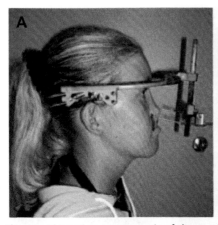 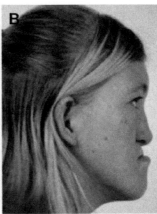 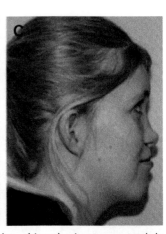

Fig. 11. Distraction osteogenesis of the maxilla. (*A*) Large advancements can be achieved using an external device. (*B*) Lateral preoperative view of maxillary retrusion. (*C*) Lateral postoperative view demonstrating important Le Fort I advancement. (*From* Phillips JH, Nish I, Daskalogiannakis J. Orthognathic surgery in cleft patients. Plast Reconstr Surg 2012;129(3):545e; with permission.)

commonly used during the consolidation period, with the aim of closing any residual open bite and maintaining the distracted occlusion.[54]

For severe maxillary deficiency Le Fort I maxillary distraction, osteogenesis offers a technique that reduces the need for bone grafts, rigid fixation systems, IMF, and blood transfusion and may decrease the length of surgical time and hospitalization.[9,27,54,61,62]

One of the drawbacks of distraction is the increased total length of treatment due to retention of the device over a 3-month period. There is also the fact that the activation arm of the internal device tends to protrude into the oral cavity, producing significant discomfort for patients. Maintenance of oral hygiene and food intake also cause patients some inconvenience.[55] Another disadvantage is the need for a second surgical stage for device removal.[54]

A challenge of using distraction techniques in orthognathic cases relates to difficulty in accurately achieving occlusal relationships. There is some ability to fine tune occlusal relationship at the time of device removal.[9] This involves the use of an interdental splint and conventional plating at the time of distractor removal.

The study of the results of the use of osteodistraction in cleft orthognathics has generally failed to show a significant difference in outcomes. No statistical difference exists in the postoperative movement achievable between single and segmental advancements in a mixed cleft population when comparing conventional orthognathic surgery with distraction osteogenesis.[55,63] There is no significant difference in the amount of anteroposterior relapse between the 2 techniques.[64] When comparing distraction to conventional

orthognathic surgery, no difference has been demonstrated with regard to the effect on speech and velopharyngeal function. No correlation was detected between the amount of maxillary advancement and the likelihood of speech and the velopharyngeal complications.[65,66]

Despite the lack of difference demonstrated between the outcomes of distraction and conventional orthognathic approaches, there is a subset of cleft patients with severe maxillary deficiency (requiring anterior advancement of >10 mm) who may benefit from distraction osteogenesis. This subgroup of patients is more prone to relapse following one-step Le Fort 1 advancement. Soft tissue restriction may contribute to the high relapse rates with one-step large advancements and to the increased incidence of velopharyngeal insufficiency.[27,52,53,67–70]

An alternative approach for patients that require movements of 18 mm or more is staged advancement. The first-stage procedure advances the maxilla as far as possible, followed by a second stage 3 to 6 months later to complete the advancement (with or without a mandibular procedure).[51]

Complications associated with distraction osteogenesis are similar to those associated with conventional orthognathic surgery, including infection and malocclusion/relapse, avascular necrosis, and oronasal fistula recurrence. Device failure and skin irritation are however specific to distractors.[54]

Virtual Surgical Planning

The use of computed tomographic scans, 3-dimensional modeling, and 3-dimensional printing can be an aid in the preoperative planning of complex cases, such as ones involving bimaxilla, multiple segments, multidirectional, and important movements or those involving distraction. When distraction has been planned, distraction devices can be carefully selected, modified, and prebent using the stereolithographic model. In this way, accurate planning of the distraction vector can be achieved. Improved access and reduced costs have seen the use of virtual surgical planning expand.

SUMMARY

Cleft orthognathic surgery is part of a complex sequence of treatments that are offered by specialist teams to manage the functional and cosmetic concerns of CL/P patients. It has considerations unique to this population and requires special planning with coordination of all members of the multidisciplinary care team. The outcomes of well-coordinated orthognathic surgery for cleft patients can be excellent; however, increased risks of relapse exist when compared with conventional patient populations. For this reason, particular surgical approaches and techniques are used to ensure the best possible results for this patient group.

REFERENCES

1. Susami T, Kuroda T, Amagasa T. Orthodontic treatment of a cleft palate patient with surgically assisted rapid maxillary expansion. Cleft Palate Craniofac J 1996;33(5):445–9.
2. Adlam DM, Yau CK, Banks P. A retrospective study of the stability of midface osteotomies in cleft lip and palate patients. Br J Oral Maxillofac Surg 1989;27(4):265–76.
3. Ewing M, Ross RB. Soft tissue response to orthognathic surgery in persons with unilateral cleft lip and palate. Cleft Palate Craniofac J 1993;30(3):320–7.
4. Hochban W, Ganss C, Austermann KH. Long-term results after maxillary advancement in patients with clefts. Cleft Palate Craniofac J 1993;30(2):237–43.
5. Good PM, Mulliken JB, Padwa BL. Frequency of Le Fort I osteotomy after repaired cleft lip and palate or cleft palate. Cleft Palate Craniofac J 2007;44(4): 396–401.
6. Mars M, James DR, Lamabadusuriya SP. The Sri Lankan cleft lip and palate project: the unoperated cleft lip and palate. Cleft Palate J 1990;27(1):3–6.
7. Herber SC, Lehman JA Jr. Orthognathic surgery in the cleft lip and palate patient. Clin Plast Surg 1993;20(4):755–68.
8. Phillips JH, Klaiman P, Delorey R, et al. Predictors of velopharyngeal insufficiency in cleft palate orthognathic surgery. Plast Reconstr Surg 2005;115(3): 681–6.
9. Phillips JH, Nish I, Daskalogiannakis J. Orthognathic surgery in cleft patients. Plast Reconstr Surg 2012; 129(3):535e–48e.
10. Posnick JC, Tompson B. Modification of the maxillary Le Fort I osteotomy in cleft-orthognathic surgery: the bilateral cleft lip and palate deformity. J Oral Maxillofac Surg 1993;51(1):2–11.
11. Aburezq H, Daskalogiannakis J, Forrest C. Management of the prominent premaxilla in bilateral cleft lip and palate. Cleft Palate Craniofac J 2006;43(1): 92–5.
12. Geraedts CT, Borstlap WA, Groenewoud JM, et al. Long-term evaluation of bilateral cleft lip and palate patients after early secondary closure and premaxilla repositioning. Int J Oral Maxillofac Surg 2007; 36(9):788–96.
13. Daskalogiannakis J, Mehta M. The need for orthognathic surgery in patients with repaired complete unilateral and complete bilateral cleft lip and palate. Cleft Palate Craniofac J 2009;46(5):498–502.
14. Ross RB. Treatment variables affecting facial growth in complete unilateral cleft lip and palate. Cleft Palate J 1987;24(1):5–77.
15. DeLuke DM, Marchand A, Robles EC, et al. Facial growth and the need for orthognathic surgery after cleft palate repair: literature review and report of 28 cases. J Oral Maxillofac Surg 1997;55(7):694–7 [discussion: 697–8].
16. Antonarakis GS, Watts G, Daskalogiannakis J. The need for orthognathic surgery in nonsyndromic patients with repaired isolated cleft palate. Cleft Palate Craniofac J 2015;52(1):e8–13.
17. Brattstrom V, McWilliam J, Larson O, et al. Craniofacial development in children with unilateral clefts of the lip, alveolus, and palate treated according to four different regimes. I. Maxillary development. Scand J Plast Reconstr Surg Hand Surg 1991; 25(3):259–67.
18. Tomanova M, Mullerova Z. Effects of primary bone grafting on facial development in patients with unilateral complete cleft lip and palate. Acta Chir Plast 1994;36(2):38–41.
19. Hathaway R, Daskalogiannakis J, Mercado A, et al. The Americleft study: an inter-center study of treatment outcomes for patients with unilateral cleft lip and palate part 2. Dental arch relationships. Cleft Palate Craniofac J 2011;48(3):244–51.
20. Semb G. Effect of alveolar bone grafting on maxillary growth in unilateral cleft lip and palate patients. Cleft Palate J 1988;25(3):288–95.
21. Daskalogiannakis J, Ross RB. Effect of alveolar bone grafting in the mixed dentition on maxillary growth in complete unilateral cleft lip and palate patients. Cleft Palate Craniofac J 1997;34(5):455–8.
22. Watts GD, Antonarakis GS, Forrest CR, et al. Single versus segmental maxillary osteotomies and long-term stability in unilateral cleft lip and palate related

malocclusion. J Oral Maxillofac Surg 2014;72(12): 2514–21.

23. Cassolato SF, Ross B, Daskalogiannakis J, et al. Treatment of dental anomalies in children with complete unilateral cleft lip and palate at SickKids hospital, Toronto. Cleft Palate Craniofac J 2009;46(2):166–72.

24. Kokich VG. Maxillary lateral incisor implants: planning with the aid of orthodontics. J Oral Maxillofac Surg 2004;62(9 Suppl 2):48–56.

25. Bell WH, Jacobs JD. Surgical-orthodontic correction of maxillary retrusion by Le Fort I osteotomy and proplast. J Maxillofac Surg 1980;8(2):84–94.

26. Persson G, Hellem S, Nord PG. Bone-plates for stabilizing Le Fort I osteotomies. J Maxillofac Surg 1986;14(2):69–73.

27. Kumar A, Gabbay JS, Nikjoo R, et al. Improved outcomes in cleft patients with severe maxillary deficiency after Le Fort I internal distraction. Plast Reconstr Surg 2006;117(5):1499–509.

28. Garib DG, Yatabe MS, Ozawa TO, et al. Alveolar bone morphology in patients with bilateral complete cleft lip and palate in the mixed dentition: cone beam computed tomography evaluation. Cleft Palate Craniofac J 2012;49(2):208–14.

29. Galante JM, Costa B, de Carvalho Carrara CF, et al. Prevalence of enamel hypoplasia in deciduous canines of patients with complete cleft lip and palate. Cleft Palate Craniofac J 2005;42(6):675–8.

30. Leshem D, Tompson B, Phillips JH. Segmental Le-Fort I surgery: turning a predicted soft-tissue failure into a success. Plast Reconstr Surg 2006;118(5): 1213–6.

31. Levy-Bercowski D, DeLeon E Jr, Stockstill JW, et al. Orthognathic cleft-surgical/orthodontic treatment. Semin Orthod 2011;17(3):197–206.

32. Miloro P. Peterson's principles of oral and maxillofacial surgery. London: BC Decker; 2004.

33. Cheng LL, Moor SL, Ho CT. Predisposing factors to dental caries in children with cleft lip and palate: a review and strategies for early prevention. Cleft Palate Craniofac J 2007;44(1):67–72.

34. Worth V, Perry R, Ireland T, et al. Are people with an orofacial cleft at a higher risk of dental caries? A systematic review and meta-analysis. Br Dent J 2017; 223(1):37–47.

35. Gaggl A, Schultes G, Kärcher H, et al. Periodontal disease in patients with cleft palate and patients with unilateral and bilateral clefts of lip, palate, and alveolus. J Periodontol 1999;70(2):171–8.

36. Posnick JC, Ricalde P. Cleft-orthognathic surgery. Clin Plast Surg 2004;31(2):315–30.

37. Jack Y, Glover A, Levy-Bercowski D. Cleft-orthognathic surgery. Philadelphia: S. Elsevier; 2008. p. 563–75.

38. Menezes R, Vieira AR. Dental anomalies as part of the cleft spectrum. Cleft Palate Craniofac J 2008; 45(4):414–9.

39. Ribeiro LL, das Neves LT, Costa B, et al. Dental development of permanent lateral incisor in complete unilateral cleft lip and palate. Cleft Palate Craniofac J 2002;39(2):193–6.

40. Carstens MH. Correction of the bilateral cleft using the sliding sulcus technique. J Craniofac Surg 2000;11(2):137–67.

41. Heliovaara A, Ranta R, Hukki J, et al. Skeletal stability of Le Fort I osteotomy in patients with isolated cleft palate and bilateral cleft lip and palate. Int J Oral Maxillofac Surg 2002;31(4):358–63.

42. Posnick JC. Orthognathic surgery for the cleft lip and palate patient. Semin Orthod 1996;2(3):205–14.

43. West R. Orthognathic srugery, an adjunct for correcting secondary cleft deformities. Oral Maxillofac Surg Clin North Am 1991;3:641–69.

44. Hoffman GR, Brennan PA. The skeletal stability of one-piece Le Fort 1 osteotomy to advance the maxilla; part 2. The influence of uncontrollable clinical variables. Br J Oral Maxillofac Surg 2004; 42(3):226–30.

45. Posnick JC, Dagys AP. Skeletal stability and relapse patterns after Le Fort I maxillary osteotomy fixed with miniplates: the unilateral cleft lip and palate deformity. Plast Reconstr Surg 1994;94(7):924–32.

46. Welch TB. Stability in the correction of dentofacial deformities: a comprehensive review. J Oral Maxillofac Surg 1989;47(11):1142–9.

47. Araujo A, Schendel SA, Wolford LM, et al. Total maxillary advancement with and without bone grafting. J Oral Surg 1978;36(11):849–58.

48. Epker BN. Superior surgical repositioning of the maxilla: long term results. J Maxillofac Surg 1981; 9(4):237–46.

49. Teuscher U, Sailer HF. Stability of Le Fort I osteotomy in class III cases with retropositioned maxillae. J Maxillofac Surg 1982;10(2):80–3.

50. Houston WJ, James DR, Jones E, et al. Le Fort I maxillary osteotomies in cleft palate cases. Surgical changes and stability. J Craniomaxillofac Surg 1989; 17(1):9–15.

51. Watts GD, Antonarakis GS, Forrest CR, et al. Is linear advancement related to relapse in unilateral cleft lip and palate orthognathic surgery? Cleft Palate Craniofac J 2015;52(6):717–23.

52. Janulewicz J, Costello BJ, Buckley MJ, et al. The effects of Le Fort I osteotomies on velopharyngeal and speech functions in cleft patients. J Oral Maxillofac Surg 2004;62(3):308–14.

53. Witzel MA, Munro IR. Velopharyngeal insufficiency after maxillary advancement. Cleft Palate J 1977; 14(2):176–80.

54. Cheung LK, Chua HD. A meta-analysis of cleft maxillary osteotomy and distraction osteogenesis. Int J Oral Maxillofac Surg 2006;35(1):14–24.

55. Cheung LK, Chua HD, Hagg MB. Cleft maxillary distraction versus orthognathic surgery: clinical

morbidities and surgical relapse. Plast Reconstr Surg 2006;118(4):996–1008 [discussion: 1009].

56. Figueroa AA, Polley JW, Friede H, et al. Long-term skeletal stability after maxillary advancement with distraction osteogenesis using a rigid external distraction device in cleft maxillary deformities. Plast Reconstr Surg 2004;114(6):1382–92 [discussion: 1393–4].

57. Baumann A, Sinko K. Importance of soft tissue for skeletal stability in maxillary advancement in patients with cleft lip and palate. Cleft Palate Craniofac J 2003;40(1):65–70.

58. Posnick JC, Taylor M. Skeletal stability and relapse patterns after Le Fort I osteotomy using miniplate fixation in patients with isolated cleft palate. Plast Reconstr Surg 1994;94(1):51–8 [discussion: 59–60].

59. Scolozzi P. Distraction osteogenesis in the management of severe maxillary hypoplasia in cleft lip and palate patients. J Craniofac Surg 2008;19(5):1199–214.

60. Doucet JC, Herlin C, Bigorre M, et al. Effects of growth on maxillary distraction osteogenesis in cleft lip and palate. J Craniomaxillofac Surg 2013;41(8):836–41.

61. Tae KC, Gong SG, Min SK, et al. Use of distraction osteogenesis in cleft palate patients. Angle Orthod 2003;73(5):602–7.

62. Yu JC, Fearon J, Havlik RJ, et al. Distraction osteogenesis of the craniofacial skeleton. Plast Reconstr Surg 2004;114(1):1E–20E.

63. Chua HD, Hagg MB, Cheung LK. Cleft maxillary distraction versus orthognathic surgery–which one is more stable in 5 years? Oral Surg Oral Med Oral Pathol Oral Radiol Endod 2010;109(6):803–14.

64. Baek SH, Lee JK, Lee JH, et al. Comparison of treatment outcome and stability between distraction osteogenesis and LeFort I osteotomy in cleft patients with maxillary hypoplasia. J Craniofac Surg 2007;18(5):1209–15.

65. Chua HD, Whitehill TL, Samman N, et al. Maxillary distraction versus orthognathic surgery in cleft lip and palate patients: effects on speech and velopharyngeal function. Int J Oral Maxillofac Surg 2010;39(7):633–40.

66. Austin SL, Mattick CR, Waterhouse PJ. Distraction osteogenesis versus orthognathic surgery for the treatment of maxillary hypoplasia in cleft lip and palate patients: a systematic review. Orthod Craniofac Res 2015;18(2):96–108.

67. Wong GB, Padwa BL. LeFort I soft tissue distraction: a hybrid technique. J Craniofac Surg 2002;13(4):572–6 [discussion: 577].

68. Kummer AW, Strife JL, Grau WH, et al. The effects of Le Fort I osteotomy with maxillary movement on articulation, resonance, and velopharyngeal function. Cleft Palate J 1989;26(3):193–9 [discussion: 199–200].

69. Okazaki K, Satoh K, Kato M, et al. Speech and velopharyngeal function following maxillary advancement in patients with cleft lip and palate. Ann Plast Surg 1993;30(4):304–11.

70. Guyette TW, Polley JW, Figueroa A, et al. Changes in speech following maxillary distraction osteogenesis. Cleft Palate Craniofac J 2001;38(3):199–205.

Pediatric Cranioplasty

Michael R. Bykowski, MD, MS[a], Jesse A. Goldstein, MD[b], Joseph E. Losee, MD[b],*

KEYWORDS

- Pediatric • Cranioplasty • Calvarial defect • Cranial defect • Skull reconstruction

KEY POINTS

- Pediatric cranioplasty has a unique set of considerations separate from adult cranioplasty, including the need for lifetime durability of the reconstruction.
- The age of the patient, location of cranial defect, and quality of the wound bed are important preoperative factors to optimize the surgical outcome.
- A well-vascularized, hearty soft tissue envelope is critical to protect the reconstruction from exposure.
- When appropriate and available, autologous bone should be used as first-line treatment.
- When autologous bone is not suitable, reconstruction of large-scale calvarial defects with porous polyethylene shows promising early outcomes.

INTRODUCTION

Cranial bone defects in children arise from various etiologies: trauma, tumor extirpation, decompressive craniectomy, infection, and congenital pathologies. Cranioplasty is any operation whose aims are to reconstruct or recontour the cranium to (1) mechanically protect the brain from direct trauma, (2) restore patient appearance, and (3) support cerebrospinal fluid dynamics and cerebral blood flow. Although these goals mirror those of the adult population, reconstructive strategies routinely practiced in adults may not be suitable for children. Furthermore, the reconstructive goals and available surgical options vary depending on the age of the child. The anatomy and physiology of the dura and rapidly expanding skull change drastically between birth and 8 years of age. Thus, reconstructive options must be tailored to the individual patient. The osteogenic properties of the dura may naturally heal cranial defects in the youngest patients (0–24 months of age), but fail to do so later in development. The absent or underdeveloped diploic space in children less than 4 years of age often renders split calvarial bone grafting

a poor reconstructive option. Additionally, it is crucial to avoid surgical management that negatively impacts normal skull and brain development. Complication rates may be higher in younger children for certain reconstructive modalities. In children less than 7 years of age, complications after hydroxyapatite cranioplasty occurred in 20.8% compared with 3.8% (range, 0%–8%) in adults and children more than 7 years old.[1,2] An additional important consideration for pediatric cranioplasty is the expected longevity of the reconstruction when compared with an adult. As such, long-term stability and resistance to extrusion are even more important in the younger patient.

SOFT TISSUE ENVELOPE

Adequate soft tissue coverage and the resolution of any infectious processes are paramount to a successful cranioplasty, be it autologous or alloplastic. The quality of the soft tissue envelope is arguably the most important factor in cranial reconstruction. Without adequate soft tissue coverage, the reconstruction can extrude,

Disclosure Statement: The authors have nothing to disclose.
[a] Department of Plastic Surgery, University of Pittsburgh Medical Center, 3550 Terrace Street, 664 Scaife Hall, Pittsburgh, PA 15261, USA; [b] Department of Plastic Surgery, Children's Hospital of Pittsburgh of University of Pittsburgh Medical Center, One Children's Hospital Drive, 4401 Penn Avenue, Faculty Pavilion, Floor 7, Pittsburgh, PA 15224, USA
* Corresponding author.
E-mail address: Joseph.losee@chp.edu

Clin Plastic Surg 46 (2019) 173–183
https://doi.org/10.1016/j.cps.2018.11.003
0094-1298/19/© 2018 Elsevier Inc. All rights reserved.

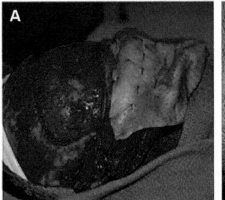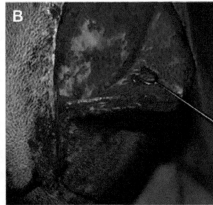

Fig. 1. Soft tissue augmentation using acellular dermal matrix (ADM). (*A*) ADM sutured to thin, scarred scalp. (*B*) ADM showing vascular ingrowth 6 months later at the time of cranioplasty.

become infected, and require further surgery. In complex calvarial defects, the soft tissues are often compromised from the initial trauma, prior scarring, chronic wounds, or infections. Defects near the vertex are further complicated by decreased perfusion. When implanting a foreign body or avascular bone graft, healthy soft tissues must be delivered to the affected area, most often using local scalp flaps and/or tissue expanded flaps. With contracted and/or inadequate soft tissues, tissue expanders, placed in a subgaleal plane, can expand native unaffected scalp. When an active infection is present, however, tissue expansion should be delayed until the successful resolution of infection. To prevent wound breakdown, a tension-free soft tissue closure is required. As an aid to achieving this goal, decreasing the projection and contour of the cranial implant and surrounding native bone can facilitate a tension-free closure without compromising the patient's appearance.[3]

Thin, compromised soft tissues can be augmented with acellular dermal matrix (ADM).[4] Incorporated ADM can add thickness to the scalp and result in an engineered vascularized scalp augmentation (**Fig. 1**). ADM can be placed at the time of cranioplasty or in a preliminary staged fashion to augment the scalp for future cranioplasty. In the setting of active infection, the defect must be rehabilitated with the removal of infected tissues and aggressive debridement of bony edges to viable, bleeding bone. To promote ADM integration, the galeal surface of the scalp is roughened with a dermabrader to create a raw and bleeding surface. A large piece of thick ADM is quilted to the galeal surface of the scalp, with the edges extending beyond the bony defect, and beneath healthy scalp tissue (see **Fig. 1**).

TIMING OF RECONSTRUCTION

The ideal timing for cranioplasty has largely been extrapolated from adult studies owing to the paucity of pediatric studies addressing this point. Cranioplasty of large cranial defects is advocated as early as possible to support perfusion of the brain and, thus, to prevent negative neurologic sequelae (eg, syndrome of the trephined). Indeed, cranioplasty provides structural support to counteract atmospheric pressure on the unprotected brain, which improves cerebral perfusion and cerebrospinal fluid dynamics.[5]

Two retrospective studies have suggested that lower complication rates are associated with early cranioplasty (performed less than 6–12 weeks after initial craniectomy).[6,7] These data, however, must be interpreted with caution owing to potential confounding factors and selection bias. For example, cranioplasty may have been delayed in sicker patients with more complex cranial defects. These recommendations, however, do not pertain to cranioplasty in the setting of infection. When the cranial defect is complicated by infection, cranioplasty should be delayed for 3 to 6 months and radiologic examinations and laboratory tests should confirm the resolution of infection before cranioplasty. When infection is present, the authors prefer delaying definitive cranioplasty for 6 months to allow for the complete resolution of infection and the plan for providing robust, vascularized soft tissue coverage. In the absence of infection, augmenting the scalp with ADM can be performed coincidentally at the time of cranioplasty.

CRANIOPLASTY MATERIALS

The ideal cranioplasty material has the following characteristics: biocompatible,   inexpensive, readily available, adequate mechanical strength, capacity for osseointegration, low infection risk, and minimal donor site morbidity. Each material has its own set of advantages and disadvantages. The clinical scenario determines the best material to use for that specific case (**Table 1**).

Autologous Bone

Autologous bone is the gold standard for cranioplasty. The specific advantages of bone include: high biocompatibility, relative availability, osteoconduction, and resistance to infection and extrusion. The use of autologous bone is inexpensive and should be used when available in sufficient quantities. Common sources of autologous bone are the bone flap from decompressive craniectomy, calvarial bone from a site distinct from the calvarial defect, rib, and iliac crest. Autologous bone integrates by osteoconduction (or creeping substitution) and depends on the healthy bony edges of the defect being in stable contact with the graft. Adequate debridement of nonviable bone edges is paramount. Bone edges of donor and recipient bones can be overlapped using a tongue-and-groove technique to maximize bone–bone contact, which promotes osteoblastic migration via creeping substitution. Thus, the larger the bone graft, the greater area of devascularized bone that depends on creeping substitution to occur before resorption. The rigid fixation of nonvascularized autologous bone grafts is crucial to minimize graft resorption and facilitate osteoconduction.[8–10]

Calvarial bone, removed at the time of a decompressive craniotomy, can be cryopreserved; however, the data demonstrates significant complications using this technique for reconstruction. Subsequent bone resorption is the most common limitation of cranioplasty using cryopreserved bone. Resorption rates of replaced bone grafts are particularly high in children and adolescents when compared with adults,[11] approaching 50% in some series and most often significant enough to require a secondary cranioplasty.[12,13] Grant and colleagues[12] found that failure of the graft strongly correlates with the size of the original skull defect. Defects of greater than 75 cm^2 had a failure rate of greater than 60%, whereas those smaller than 75 cm^2 were associated with no failures. In addition to defect size, the timing of reconstruction impacts surgical success. Resorption of cryopreserved bone is significantly greater (42%) when delayed beyond 6 weeks compared with 14% when performed earlier.[6]

Calvarial bone grafts from unaffected skull, rib, and iliac crest are common donor sites, but are of limited usefulness in the setting of large defects (especially rib and iliac crest), particularly in the young child. Calvarial bone for reconstruction has the advantage of replacing "like with like," being in close proximity to the defect, and can be harvested as particulate bone graft, split-thickness bone graft, full-thickness bone grafts (ie, switch cranioplasty), or as a combination of split- or full-thickness grafts and particulate graft. Particulate bone graft can be harvested using the Safescraper (Osteogenics Biomedical; Lubbock, TX) or a Hudson brace.[14] One limitation of particulate bone alone is that it cannot be used as a structural graft.

For children younger than 4 to 5 years of age, the skull is a trilaminar structure with a central soft cancellous diploic space. Thus, split-thickness bone grafts can be used in this population. Traditional teaching, however, is that cranial bone cannot be meaningfully split before the age of 3 years because of the lack of a well-developed diploic space. This dictum has subsequently been challenged in small bone defects in patient with craniosynostosis.[15,16]

Split-thickness bone grafts have reduced thickness and stability compared with full-thickness bone grafts. The exchange cranioplasty is an option, whereby the existing defect is repaired with a full-thickness structural calvarial graft taken from an unaffected area of the cranium to repair the osseous defect. The donor site, which has physiologically normal dura, pericranium, and healthy overlying scalp, is then covered with particulate bone graft harvested from the endocortex of the structural graft (or ectocortex of intact adjacent cranium). Several technical issues should be considered when implementing this technique. First, the graft should be harvested at a low drill speed to avoid thermal injury to the bone. The surgeon must take into consideration the kerf of the drill bit—that is, a drill bit no larger than 1 cm should be used to maximize the amount of structural bone graft while limiting the donor defect size. When also using adjacent ectocortical bone, thick cranial bone (eg, parietal bone) is preferred. The particulate bone graft should be placed over the donor site dura to a thickness of at least 4 to 5 mm (but ideally to the thickness of surrounding bone to maximize bony contact and healing). Fibrin glue can be used to help prevent bone particulate from dislodging when redraping the pericranium and scalp soft tissues. Using this technique, Rogers and Greene[17] reviewed 20 cases with an average defect size of 85 cm^2, and found that 15 of the 20 had complete healing and the size of the defects decreased by an average of 96%. As one might expect, the largest initial calvarial defects resulted in the largest persistent

Table 1
Characteristics of cranioplasty materials

Cranioplasty Type	Precision	Durability	Osseointegration	Growth Potential	Donor Site Morbidity	Cost	Infection Risk
Autologous							
Bone graft	Difficult to contour/shape	Potential to resorb	Excellent	Excellent	Significant with large defects	Minimal	Low
Alloplastic							
Titanium	Good precision with potential to customize	Rigid	Poor	Potential restriction	None	High	Low but relatively high extrusion rate
PMMA	Good precision with potential to customize	Brittle	Limited	Potential restriction	None	Low	High when communicates with sinus
HA	Cement form is moldable	Brittle when used alone	Good	Potential restriction	None	Low	High when communicates with sinus
Medpor	Good precision with potential to customize	Rigid	Poor	Potential restriction	None	High	Low
PEEK	Good precision with potential to customize	Rigid	Poor	Limited data	None	High	Limited data

Abbreviations: HA, hydroxyapatite; PEEK, polyaryl ether ether ketone; PMMA, polymethylmethacrylate.

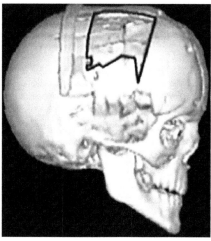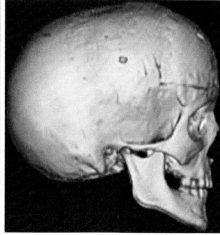

Fig. 2. Preoperative planning of custom-made porous polyethylene implant for hemicalvarial defect in a 4-year-old patient using computer-assisted design and manufacturing (CAD/CAM).

bony defect (ranging from 11 to 27 cm^2). Similar to all bone grafts, survival of the particulate and structural grafts depends on the health and vascularity of the surrounding tissue bed. Thus, exchange cranioplasty should be avoided in areas of infected, damaged, or scarred wound beds. Last, although the donor defects healed to near completion (98%) in this small clinical series, a disadvantage is the creation of a secondary calvarial defect.

Potential donor site morbidity can be avoided by using commercially available demineralized bone matrix (DBX) as a substrate. The DBX collagen scaffold allows for osteoconduction and the retained bone morphogenetic protein provides osteoinduction. DBX can be combined with bioresorbable mesh in a bilaminate fashion, that is, a sandwich cranioplasty. More specifically, a bilaminate construct is created with bioresorbable mesh placed endocranially on the dura, layered with DBX with or without particulate bone graft, and buttressed with an outer layer of bioresorbable mesh.[18] This technique provides an initial rigid and protective reconstruction that is, replaced by bone during the natural resorption of the mesh (**Fig. 2**). The rigid sandwich construct of polylactic acid/polyglycolic acid plates resists the deformational forces of the overlying scalp and underlying pulsatile dura while preserving the space filled with DBX mix. This method can be used successfully in reconstructing donor defects (eg, exchange cranioplasty) or primary defects (eg, skull expansion), when there is healthy, nonscarred soft tissues to provide a vascularized bed for reconstruction. This technique has been proven less successful in the altered environment of a scarred bed.[18] Once integrated, however,

autologous bone has minimal infection and exposure risk.

Alloplastic Materials

The development of alloplastic cranioplasty has evolved from the limitations and morbidities of autologous bone grafts. If the skull defect is large or donor bone is inadequate, then alloplastic materials can be considered. These materials should be biocompatible, rigid, incorporate into surrounding bone, and present a low infection risk. Each material discussed herein has its specific advantages and disadvantages. A potential disadvantage of using alloplastic materials for pediatric cranioplasty is the theoretic risk of growth restriction. The degree of growth restriction—if it does indeed occur—would depend on the patient's age and growth potential. Cranial growth is nearly complete around the age of 6 years; thus, the theoretic impact on growth restriction should be minimal when cranioplasty is performed beyond this time. No adequate long-term pediatric studies have yet been published to either support or negate this theory of growth restriction. However, the authors have a series of patients (presented elsewhere in this article) who have undergone alloplastic reconstruction with porous polyethylene at a very young age, now with midterm data suggesting that growth restriction has not occurred.

Titanium

Titanium is often mixed with aluminum and vanadium to create an alloy that is lightweight, rigid, able to be contoured, relatively biocompatible/inert (even when exposed), heat resistant, and radiolucent. As discussed, a theoretic

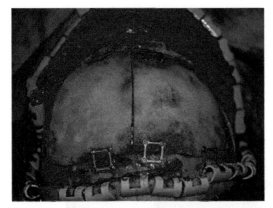

Fig. 3. Case 1. Porous polyethylene implant for a bifrontal defect in a 3.2-year-old patient, split intraoperatively for better fit.

disadvantage often cited related to titanium cranioplasty is the potential for growth restriction, although further long-term growth data are scarce in the pediatric population.

In general, titanium cranioplasty is not well-studied in the pediatric population. Ma and colleagues,[19] however, recently reported their experience with 33 pediatric patients who underwent titanium cranioplasty. There were 2 cases of late exposure of titanium mesh. Long-term follow-up was not available for all patients, which is necessary to demonstrate stable reconstruction with implant extrusion. Titanium has also been used as a scaffold upon which acrylic or ceramic alloplastics are applied to optimize intraoperative contouring and aesthetic outcomes.

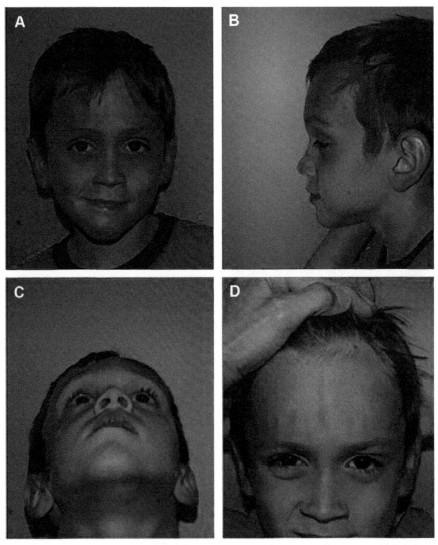

Fig. 4. Case 1. Postoperative result at 9 years of age, 6.7 years after cranioplasty. Frontal (*A*), lateral (*B*), and worm's eye views (*C*). See preserved frontalis function and visible midline indentation from implant splitting (*D*).

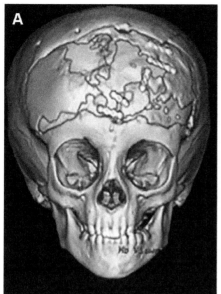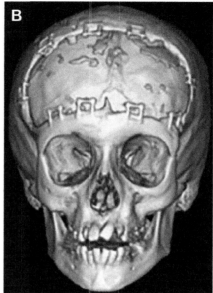

Fig. 5. Case 1. Three-dimensional reconstruction of a computed tomography scan at 3 years of age, showing failed autologous bone reconstruction (*A*). Three-dimensional reconstruction at 9 years of age with porous polyethylene implant in place (*B*). Notice normal-appearing craniofacial growth.

Finally, in young children with an underdeveloped diploic space, monocortical screws used for implant fixation can migrate intracranially and pose a potential risk of penetrating the underlying dura and cerebral cortex.[20] Translocation of metallic hardware can result from normal skull growth, which in part occurs as the endocranial bone surface resorbs and bone is deposited on the ectocranial surface.

Acrylics

Polymethylmethacrylate (PMMA) is a readily available and inexpensive polymer with strength and biocompatibility profiles similar to that of bone.

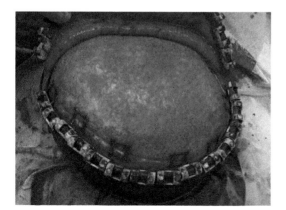

Fig. 6. Case 2. Porous polyethylene implant for a hemicranial defect in a 21-month-old patient.

PMMA has limited ability for osseointegration. PMMA is often packaged as a powdered form and is mixed on demand to form a malleable putty, which hardens into a form-stable solid within 4 to 6 minutes of polymerization. Of note, this reaction is exothermic and can burn the dura and surrounding tissues. When used as a standalone cranioplasty material, PMMA can be brittle. To augment its strength, PMMA has been used in combination with titanium. Although PMMA is somewhat resistant to infection, it should be avoided in frontal cranioplasty when there is a high potential of nasal/frontal sinus continuity. Marchac and Greensmith[21] reported an infection rate of 45.5% when PMMA was in continuity with a sinus compared with only 1.9% when not continuous with a sinus. Long-term outcomes with PMMA are favorable and the complication rates remain low, but only in the absence of postoperative radiotherapy, large cranial defect, involvement of the frontal sinus, and the presence of prior infection.[22]

Ceramics

Calcium phosphates resemble the inorganic matrix of bone. Similar to bone, calcium phosphates have osteoconductive properties and are biocompatible. Calcium phosphates are derived from naturally occurring corals, but may also be synthesized in the laboratory. There are 2 main varieties of hydrated calcium phosphate (hydroxyapatite

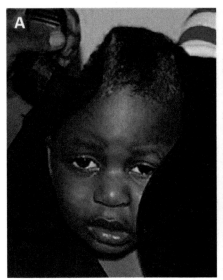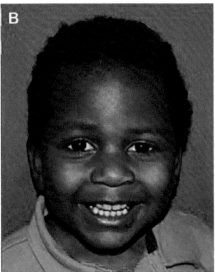

Fig. 7. Case 2. Patient before (*A*) and after cranioplasty (*B*), with dramatic neurologic improvement.

[HA]) preparations for use in bone applications: ceramics and cements.

Ceramic forms of HA are difficult to shape and can be brittle, fracturing in the operating room or after trauma. Unlike ceramic forms, HA cements are moldable, which allows for intraoperative contouring. These implants are burdened with high complication rates when there is communication with sinuses. In a study over 20 years and with more than 2500 (adult and pediatric) patients treated with custom HA implants, the infection rate was approximately 2%, with a late posttraumatic fracture rate of just over 1.5% in adults and 4% in children.[23] For carbonated calcium phosphate cement, the risk of infection when exposed to sinuses is high. Owing to its fragility, the use of carbonated calcium phosphate cement should be limited to small defects and as onlay grafts with a contouring cranioplasty, rather than for full-thickness skull reconstruction.[24,25]

Plastics

The advantages of plastics include inert reaction, durable construction, nondegradable stability, customizable properties, and a porous framework, which allows for theoretic vascular and bony ingrowth. The 2 most popular plastic cranioplasty materials are porous polyethylene (Medpor) and polyaryl ether ether ketone (PEEK). Porous polyethylene has been popularized as a material resistant to infection.

When autologous bone is not a reasonable first-line option, the authors prefer porous polyethylene for large-scale calvarial reconstruction; they have

reported on a series of young children followed in their craniofacial center.[26] Indeed, in the authors' initial experience, large defect Medpor cranioplasty was originally planned to be a temporizing measure to bridge pediatric patients to the definitive cranioplasty, awaiting growth and the development of a more robust diploic space, suitable for autologous bone reconstruction with split calvarial bone graft. The high-density polyethylene is engineered to produce a porous framework that allows for soft tissue ingrowth. Subsequent studies have suggested that porous polyethylene is limited in its ability to allow osteoconduction.[27] These implants are commercially available and can be prefabricated. Moreover, porous polyethylene can be contoured on the table with tailoring of the custom implant with a scalpel to achieve the best inset. The main advantage of porous polyethylene is its low complication rate, which has been attributed to the avidity for vascular ingrowth.[28] In 2012, the authors reported a series of pediatric patients in which 9 patients underwent cranioplasty of large-scale defects (mean size, 152 cm²).[26] There were no infections or implant extrusions. However, the mean follow-up at the time was short at only 3.6 months. These patients have been followed and 3 additional patients have been added to the series with longer follow-up averaging 5.1 years. Eight defects are hemicranial and 4 are bifrontal. One patient was a 2-year-old boy with no prior reconstruction and the other 11 patients had failed replaced cryopreserved bone flaps. Before Medpor cranioplasty, 50% of patients had neurosurgical courses complicated by bone and/or shunt

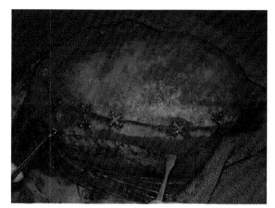

Fig. 8. Case 3. Porous polyethylene implant for a hemicranial defect in a 4.1-year-old patient.

infections and multiple interventions. Definitive cranioplasty was delayed until infection had resolved with directed antibiotic treatment and appropriate debridements. With more than 5 years of follow-up, 11 of the 12 patients (92%) had stable implants with no soft tissue or implant-related complications. One patient had their implant removed 5 years after cranioplasty after the inadvertent placement of a ventriculoperitoneal shunt inserted through the implant and subsequent development of a shunt infection. Before this event, there were no infectious, growth, or soft tissue complications. In this series, the soft tissues overlying the implant are supple and mobile with no evidence of soft tissue thinning or implant exposure. As with all children with thin soft tissues, hardware palpability is an issue and, occasionally, the hardware can be visible. Thus far, this has not

become a medical or cosmetic concern for the patients or families. **Figs. 3–10** demonstrate 3 cases of Medpor cranioplasty.

Cranial growth has been followed meticulously and has been challenging to accurately assess in the setting of prior neurotrauma. In the small series of patients, those without underlying significant brain injury have demonstrated normal skull growth velocity, despite having undergone large scale alloplastic cranioplasty. Eight patients had long-term follow-up computed tomography scans (mean follow-up, 6.5 years; range, 5.5–8.1 years). Compared with age-matched skeletally normal children,[29] cranial length and width measurements were within normal ranges for 7 of 8 children (88%). Of note, the other child (see **Fig. 7**), who initially had significant neurologic deficits that improved after cranioplasty, still has persistent diffuse volume and density loss of the right brain hemisphere.

PEEK material is one of the newest materials to be used in pediatric cranioplasty. PEEK's elasticity and energy-absorbing properties are closer to that of bone when compared with titanium.[30] Because of its relative newness, long-term data in a substantial cohort are unavailable. A recent study reports early follow-up of 33 months for 28 PEEK implants.[31] The implant failure rate was 21%, defined as any subsequent surgery performed to remove the cranioplasty implant, replacing it with a new implant because of infection, dislodgement, or unacceptable cosmesis. PEEK, however, does not integrate with bone, nor is it porous enough to allow for soft tissue ingrowth; therefore, it must rely on a tight approximation to bone.

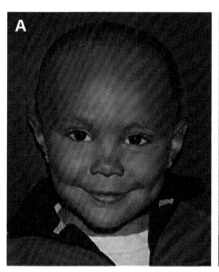
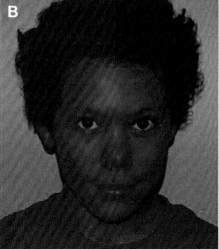

Fig. 9. Case 3. Patient at 5 years of age, 1 year after cranioplasty (*A*), and at 12 years of age, 7.8 years after cranioplasty (*B*).

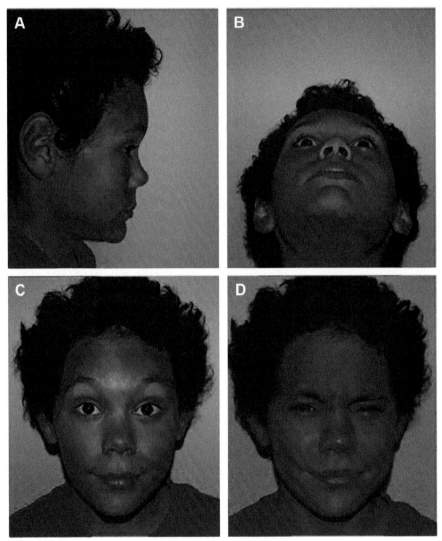

Fig. 10. Case 3. Notice adequate forehead projection and contour in lateral (*A*) and worm's eye views (*B*). Preserved and symmetric function of forehead muscles (*C, D*).

Indeed, Bowers and colleagues[31] noted that the only factor that was associated with failure was a bone-implant gap of more than 6 mm.

SUMMARY

There is a wide range of options for pediatric calvarial reconstruction. The specific technique used for cranioplasty depends on the age of the patient, location of cranial defect, the quality of the wound bed, and the availability of potential autologous bony donor sites. A well-vascularized, hearty soft tissue envelope is critical to protect from exposure of the reconstruction. When appropriate and available, autologous bone should be used for reconstruction. When autologous bone is not suitable, however, reconstruction of large-scale calvarial defects with Medpor shows promising early outcomes. Because the cranioplasty must last the subsequent decades of the child's lifetime, long-term data are still needed before definitive recommendations can be finalized.

REFERENCES

1. Stefini R, Esposito G, Zanotti B, et al. Use of "custom made" porous hydroxyapatite implants for cranioplasty: postoperative analysis of complications in 1549 patients. Surg Neurol Int 2013;4:12.
2. Frassanito P, Tamburrini G, Massimi L, et al. Postmarketing surveillance of CustomBone Service implanted in children under 7 years old. Acta Neurochir (Wien) 2015;157(1):115–21.

3. Nout E, Mommaerts MY. Considerations in computer-aided design for inlay cranioplasty: technical note. Oral Maxillofac Surg 2018;22(1):65–9.

4. Kinsella CR Jr, Grunwaldt LJ, Cooper GM, et al. Scalp reconstruction: regeneration with acellular dermal matrix. J Craniofac Surg 2010;21(2):605–7.

5. Mah JK, Kass RA. The impact of cranioplasty on cerebral blood flow and its correlation with clinical outcome in patients underwent decompressive craniectomy. Asian J Neurosurg 2016;11(1):15–21.

6. Piedra MP, Thompson EM, Selden NR, et al. Optimal timing of autologous cranioplasty after decompressive craniectomy in children. J Neurosurg Pediatr 2012;10(4):268–72.

7. Chang V, Hartzfeld P, Langlois M, et al. Outcomes of cranial repair after craniectomy. J Neurosurg 2010; 112(5):1120–4.

8. Ono I, Gunji H, Kaneko F, et al. Treatment of extensive cranial bone defects using computer-designed hydroxyapatite ceramics and periosteal flaps. Plast Reconstr Surg 1993;92(5):819–30.

9. DeLacure MD. Physiology of bone healing and bone grafts. Otolaryngol Clin North Am 1994;27(5): 859–74.

10. Citardi MJ, Friedman CD. Nonvascularized autogenous bone grafts for craniofacial skeletal augmentation and replacement. Otolaryngol Clin North Am 1994;27(5):891–910.

11. Fan MC, Wang QL, Sun P, et al. Cryopreservation of autologous cranial bone flaps for cranioplasty: a large sample retrospective study. World Neurosurg 2018;109:e853–9.

12. Grant GA, Jolley M, Ellenbogen RG, et al. Failure of autologous bone-assisted cranioplasty following decompressive craniectomy in children and adolescents. J Neurosurg 2004;100(2 Suppl Pediatrics): 163–8.

13. Piitulainen JM, Kauko T, Aitasalo KM, et al. Outcomes of cranioplasty with synthetic materials and autologous bone grafts. World Neurosurg 2015; 83(5):708–14.

14. Greene AK, Mulliken JB, Proctor MR, et al. Pediatric cranioplasty using particulate calvarial bone graft. Plast Reconstr Surg 2008;122(2):563–71.

15. Vercler CJ, Sugg KB, Buchman SR. Split cranial bone grafting in children younger than 3 years old: debunking a surgical myth. Plast Reconstr Surg 2014;133(6):822e–7e.

16. Steinbok P, Seal SK, Courtemanche DJ. Split calvarial bone grafting in patients less than 1 year of age: technical note and use in craniofacial surgery for craniosynostosis. Childs Nerv Syst 2011;27(7): 1149–52.

17. Rogers GF, Greene AK. Autogenous bone graft: basic science and clinical implications. J Craniofac Surg 2012;23(1):323–7.

18. Chao MT, Jiang S, Smith D, et al. Demineralized bone matrix and resorbable mesh bilaminate cranioplasty: a novel method for reconstruction of large-scale defects in the pediatric calvaria. Plast Reconstr Surg 2009;123(3):976–82.

19. Ma IT, Symon MR, Bristol RE, et al. Outcomes of titanium mesh cranioplasty in pediatric patients. J Craniofac Surg 2018;29(1):99–104.

20. Duke BJ, Mouchantat RA, Ketch LL, et al. Transcranial migration of microfixation plates and screws. Case report. Pediatr Neurosurg 1996;25(1):31–4 [discussion: 35].

21. Marchac D, Greensmith A. Long-term experience with methylmethacrylate cranioplasty in craniofacial surgery. J Plast Reconstr Aesthet Surg 2008;61(7): 744–52 [discussion: 753].

22. Blum KS, Schneider SJ, Rosenthal AD. Methyl methacrylate cranioplasty in children: long-term results. Pediatr Neurosurg 1997;26(1):33–5.

23. Stefini R, Zanotti B, Nataloni A, et al. The efficacy of custom-made porous hydroxyapatite prostheses for cranioplasty: evaluation of postmarketing data on 2697 patients. J Appl Biomater Funct Mater 2015; 13(2):e136–44.

24. Gilardino MS, Cabiling DS, Bartlett SP. Long-term follow-up experience with carbonated calcium phosphate cement (Norian) for cranioplasty in children and adults. Plast Reconstr Surg 2009;123(3): 983–94.

25. Zins JE, Moreira-Gonzalez A, Papay FA. Use of calcium-based bone cements in the repair of large, full-thickness cranial defects: a caution. Plast Reconstr Surg 2007;120(5):1332–42.

26. Lin AY, Kinsella CR Jr, Rottgers SA, et al. Custom porous polyethylene implants for large-scale pediatric skull reconstruction: early outcomes. J Craniofac Surg 2012;23(1):67–70.

27. Tark WH, Yoon IS, Rah DK, et al. Osteoconductivity of porous polyethylene in human skull. J Craniofac Surg 2012;23(1):78–80.

28. Liu JK, Gottfried ON, Cole CD, et al. Porous polyethylene implant for cranioplasty and skull base reconstruction. Neurosurg Focus 2004;16(3).

29. Waitzman AA, Posnick JC, Armstrong DC, et al. Craniofacial skeletal measurements based on computed tomography: part II. Normal values and growth trends. Cleft Palate Craniofac J 1992;29(2): 118–28.

30. Lethaus B, Safi Y, ter Laak-Poort M, et al. Cranioplasty with customized titanium and PEEK implants in a mechanical stress model. J Neurotrauma 2012;29(6):1077–83.

31. Bowers CA, McMullin JH, Brimley C, et al. Minimizing bone gaps when using custom pediatric cranial implants is associated with implant success. J Neurosurg Pediatr 2015;16(4):439–44.

State-of-the-Art Hypertelorism Management

Sameer Shakir, MD[a], Ian C. Hoppe, MD[a],
Jesse A. Taylor, MD[b],*

KEYWORDS

- Orbital hypertelorism • Interorbital hypertelorism • Facial bipartition • Box osteotomy
- Chula technique • MOCUT

KEY POINTS

- *Orbital* hypertelorism represents lateralization of the orbits, meaning increased interorbital and outer orbital distances.
- *Interorbital* hypertelorism represents a failure of medial orbital wall medialization in the setting of normally positioned lateral orbital walls.
- The etiology and type of hypertelorism influence selection of an operative procedure, whereas the severity of deformity dictates surgical need.
- Choice of surgical procedure is dictated by anatomic considerations such as degree of orbital hypertelorism, midfacial proportions, and occlusal status.

EMBRYOLOGIC DEVELOPMENT

The delicate sequence of craniofacial development demonstrates that the "face predicts the brain."[1] Facial development occurs between gestational weeks 4 and 8, during which time the midface develops immediately anterior to the forebrain. Paired nasal placodes and maxillary processes migrate medially as the frontonasal process shifts cephalically. As the frontonasal prominence narrows to become the nasal root and bridge, the optic placodes move laterally to medially toward the midline. Failure of the frontonasal process to narrow prevents medialization of the eyes, resulting in congenital anomalies of the forehead, nose, and orbits. The term "orbital hypertelorism" was credited to Paul Tessier[2] in 1974 to describe a congenital failure of the orbits to medialize, leading to an increased distance between the orbits.

DEFINITIONS

David Greig[3] coined the phrase "ocular hypertelorism" in 1924 to describe a craniofacial deformity associated with "a great breadth between the eyes." Serving as a contrast to Greig's[3] concept of "ocular hypertelorism," Tessier[2] reasoned that true hypertelorism represented a congenital divergence of the bony orbits (ie, both medial and lateral walls) and not simply an increased interpupillary distance that could result from various acquired injuries. Van der Meulen and Vaandrager[4] further refined the term to describe a "true lateralization of orbits," as determined by an abnormally obtuse angle created along the axes of the lateral orbital walls. Hence, true orbital hypertelorism represents increased interorbital and outer orbital distances. Tessier[2] attributed true hypertelorism to etiologically and pathogenetically heterogeneous causes, including (1) frontonasal malformation,

Disclosure: The authors have nothing to disclose.
[a] Division of Plastic Surgery, University of Pennsylvania, 3400 Civic Center Blvd, Philadelphia, PA 19104, USA;
[b] Division of Plastic Surgery, The Children's Hospital of Philadelphia, 3401 Civic Center Blvd, Philadelphia, PA 19104, USA
* Corresponding author.
E-mail address: jataylor@gmail.com

Clin Plastic Surg 46 (2019) 185–195
https://doi.org/10.1016/j.cps.2018.11.004
0094-1298/19/© 2018 Elsevier Inc. All rights reserved.

(2) craniofrontonasal dysplasia, (3) paramedian craniofacial clefts, and (4) encephalocele. Tessier's[2] classification schema in adults used the interorbital distance, as measured from dacryon to dacryon, to define first-degree (30–34 mm), second-degree (34–40 mm), and third-degree (>40 mm) deformities. He further reasoned that the interorbital distance and overall shape of the orbits determined the surgical consequences. Tan and Mulliken[5] graded hypertelorism in children based on standard deviation (SD) from age-matched and gender-matched data: (1) first degree (2.0–4.0 SDs above the norm), (2) second degree (4.1–8.0 SDs), and (3) third degree (>8.1 SDs).

Interorbital hypertelorism, unlike ocular hypertelorism, represents a failure of medial orbital wall medialization in the setting of normally positioned lateral orbital walls. Van der Meulen and Vaandrager[4] differentiated this form of hypertelorism from the orbital variant based on the angle between the lateral orbital walls on computed tomography (CT) axial imaging; interorbital hypertelorism was radiographically defined as an angle of 90°, whereas orbital hypertelorism represented a more obtuse angle. Embryologically, this represents abnormal development following medialization of the orbits, thereby either inhibiting primary medialization or causing increased secondary lateralization of the medial orbits.[6] This hypertelorism iteration is most commonly found in patients with frontoethmoidal meningoencephaloceles. Interestingly, it is the authors' experience that interorbital hypertelorism is commonly found as a secondary deformity after primary surgery for ocular hypertelorism.

HISTORY

The earliest report of attempted orbital hypertelorism reconstruction dates to 1950. Webster and Deming[7] aimed to reverse the appearance of the "bifid nose" through soft tissue corrections of the "epicanthal folds, wide-set eyebrows, and broad nose with bulbous tip." Between 1959 and 1962, Converse and colleagues[8] and Smith described an extracranial approach used in 3 patients to medially relocate the medial canthus and a portion of the medial orbital wall.[9] Schmid[10] then successfully medialized the circumferential orbit with the addition of an orbital roof osteotomy by exploiting a patient's hyperpneumatized frontal sinuses in 1968. In reviewing these early techniques, Tessier and colleagues[11] rightfully concluded that these early extracranial techniques were "doomed to fail," as they did not reposition the orbital walls, periorbita, or globes and required a high cribiform plate to permit safe osteotomy without intracranial

injury. Interestingly, his conclusions remain true, as extracranial approaches are only reserved for mild cases of hypertelorism and only to correct telecanthus. They instead proposed a radical intracranial approach based on the principles that (1) devascularization and reshaping of the craniofacial skeleton does not affect its viability, (2) complete mobilization and repositioning of the orbits does not affect vision, and (3) combined intracranial and extracranial surgery produces drastic changes to the craniofacial skeleton.[11]

As the story goes in the Parisian Hôpital Foch in 1962, Paul Tessier asked his neurosurgeon Gérard Guyot if the bony orbits could be medialized via an intracranial approach.[12] He famously replied, "Pourquoi pas?" (Why not?), now eternalized as the moniker for the International Society of Craniofacial Surgery. Tessier[2] subsequently published his series of 52 patients beginning in 1962 who underwent medialization of the bony orbits via an intracranial approach, paving the way for a surgical breakthrough in the treatment of orbital hypertelorism.

CLASSIFICATION

Mulliken and colleagues[5] reviewed 90 clinical cases of hypertelorism based on the aforementioned etiologies and concluded (1) etiology and type (ie, interorbital vs true orbital) influence selection of an operative procedure and (2) severity (ie, degree) dictates surgical need. For example, a child with orbital hypertelorism would benefit from intracranial translocation of the orbits versus a child with interorbital hypertelorism, but only if the deformity was second or third degree. In his analysis, 30 (33%) presented with frontonasal malformations, 18 (20%) with craniofrontonasal dysplasia, 10 (11%) with median and paramedian clefts, 6 (7%) with encephaloceles, and 26 (29%) with miscellaneous chromosomal or syndromic disorders.

Frontonasal Malformations

Frontonasal malformations encompass the terms median cleft face syndrome, frontonasal syndrome, and frontonasal dysplasia. These malformations do not represent a single developmental localized defect, but rather present as a heterogeneous category of variable facial appearances. They are defined by symmetric hypertelorism associated with variable midline facial defects including (1) bifid nose, (2) median cleft upper lip and premaxilla, (3) median cleft palate, (4) widow's peak, and (5) anterior cranium bifidum occultum. There are no documented reports of familial transmission or gender predominance.

Craniofrontonasal Dysplasia

Unlike frontonasal malformations, craniofrontonasal dysplasia (CFND) represents a rare familial craniofacial syndrome that is sex-linked with an unusual pattern of inheritance. There is a strong gender preference favoring female patients who invariably present with more severe phenotypes than their male counterparts. Coronal synostosis (either unilateral or bilateral) represents the primary feature of CFND in addition to a variety of frontonasal deformities including a broad nasal bridge and tip and down-slanting palpebral fissures. The orbital hypertelorism found in CFND may be asymmetric. Unique extracranial features include thick "frizzy" hair, shoulder and hip girdle abnormalities, and longitudinal ridging of finger or toenails. Additional associated anomalies include cleft lip or palate, high-arched palate, maxillary hypoplasia, strabismus, soft tissue syndactyly of the fingers and toes, and broad thumb or great toe. Surgery involves craniosynostosis correction usually achieved by fronto-orbital advancement during infancy and later orbital translocation. Facial bipartition may be used to simultaneously reposition the bony orbits and correct malocclusion, given the hypoplastic midface and misshapen maxilla, facial bipartition.

Paramedian Facial Clefts and the Tessier Classification System

Paul Tessier[13] introduced the Tessier classification system of facial clefts based on his clinical examination and surgical experience in 1976. He first described "clefting" as a process involving "interruption of either soft tissue or skeleton" and used the eyelid and orbit as his frames of reference, as these structures are common to both the cranium and face. He recognized that facial clefts are found around the orbit and eyes and jaws and lips, with the skeletal providing more consistent landmarks compared with the overlying soft tissues. The classification system uses a numbering system (no. 0–14) with 8 time-zones to describe 15 locations for clefts. For orientation purposes, his system divides the orbit into 2 hemispheres with clefts running downward from the lower lid (no. 0–6) classified as facial (southbound) and clefts running upward from the upper lid (no. 7–14) as cranial (northbound). The median facial dysraphia serves as the no. 0 with subsequent clefts numbered in relation to this zero line. For example, the midline widening demonstrated in frontonasal dysplasia corresponds to a 0 to 14 cleft. Interestingly, Tessier had yet to see a patient with a no. 9 cleft when formulating his system.[13] Clinically, patients with facial clefting present with facial and cranial clefts equaling 14, which allows for accurate representation of the clefting

process above and below the orbit. In the series of Tan and Mulliken,[5] patients with facial clefts presented with asymmetric orbital hypertelorism and cranial cleft elements.

Encephaloceles

An encephalocele can be defined as a herniation of meninges (meningocele) through a congenital bony defect with or without brain (encephalomengingocele). The internal defect lies at the junction of the frontal and ethmoidal bones, whereas the external or facial defect can vary. Mahatumarat and colleagues[14] described their classification system based on characteristics of the external bone defect including type and location: (1) nasofrontal (between nasal and frontal bones), (2) nasoethmoidal (between nasal bones and cartilages), (3) naso-orbital (through medial orbital wall), (4) combined (nasoethmoidal and naso-orbital coexist), and (5) abortive (external bone defect unidentifiable). Associated findings include telecanthus, epiphora, dacryocystitis, and other facial and ocular deformities. Although the overall incidence is rare, encephaloceles are more common in Southern and Southeast Asia, with the highest incidence of frontoethmoidal encephalomeningoceles occurring in 1:3500 to 1:6000 births annually in these regions.[14] It should be noted that encephaloceles can occur as a secondary feature in frontonasal malformations, craniofrontonasal dysplasia, and paramedian facial clefting.

Miscellaneous

Mulliken and colleagues classified 26 (29%) patients with hypertelorism as stemming from a miscellaneous etiology, which again emphasizes the heterogeneity of hypertelorism as a physical examination finding found in a variety of craniofacial disorders. Interestingly, first-degree and second-degree interorbital hypertelorism was noted in 7 patients with cleft lip and palate, further corroborating prior reports.[15] These etiologies include bilateral cleft lip and palate, chromosomal abnormalities (ie, trisomy 13–15), and several named syndromes (ie, Turner, Robinow, Teebi, Aarskog, Axenfeld, and oculoauriculofrontonasal). They observed symmetric hypertelorism in all patients but 3 patients who presented with duplicated maxilla, oculoauriculofrontonasal syndrome, or ophthalmofrontonasal syndrome.[5]

SURGICAL APPROACHES

Surgical aims guiding the correction of hypertelorism include (1) medialization of the orbits, (2) nasal reconstruction, and (3) correction of midface

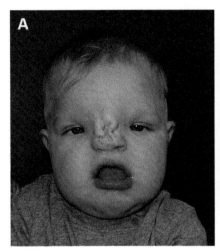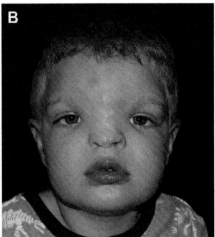

Fig. 1. (*A*) Ten-month-old with cutis gyrate. (*B*) Following excision of cutis gyrate.

abnormalities, if applicable. Correction has consequently evolved from historical extracranial or subcranial approaches to the modern-day intracranial approaches popularized by Tessier.[11,16,17] We highlight the extracranial Chula technique to contrast with the intracranial 4-wall box osteotomy, facial bipartition, and medial orbital composite-unit translocation (MOCUT) procedures used at our institution (**Fig. 1**).

Factors affecting surgical decision-making include age, type of hypertelorism (ie, interorbital vs orbital hypertelorism), etiology, and midface abnormalities (ie, occlusion). Although variation exists that requires individual treatment plans for each patient, we generally recommend the following algorithm: (1) MOCUT when the lateral walls are in anatomic position and the medial walls are lateralized (ie, interorbital hypertelorism), (2) 4-wall "box" osteotomy when true orbital hypertelorism exists and the midface is not deficient, and (3) symmetric or asymmetric facial bipartition with distraction when true orbital hypertelorism exists and the midface is deficient with a V-shaped upper occlusal plane. Sometimes a degree of cutis gyrata can be present over the nasal dorsum, necessitating an excision at the time of bony reconstruction or before this for aesthetic reasons (see **Fig. 1**).

Interorbital Hypertelorism

Chula technique
In 1991, Mahatumarat and colleagues[18] introduced the Chula technique as a single-stage extracranial procedure for the reconstruction of interorbital hypertelorism due to encephaloceles, specifically frontoethmoidal encephalomeningoceles in children as young as 3 months (**Fig. 2**). Named after the Thai King Chulalongkorn, this

nasocoronal technique involves an extracranial T-shaped osteotomy of the superomedial orbital rim and medial orbital walls, which is subsequently narrowed and fixated in place medially.[14] The surgical approach involves a traditional bicoronal scalp flap in combination with a lambda-type curvilinear incision over the nasal encephalocele skin to (1) access the encephalocele, (2) dissect the herniated glial tissue and identify the internal bony defect, (3) secure the medial canthal tendons with wire for later canthopexy. and (4) resect redundant skin. After removal of the T-shaped bony element, any dural repairs are repaired primarily or with pericranial flaps. The internal bony defect is reconstructed with an inlay tantalum mesh prosthetic, whereas the narrowed T-shaped segment is replaced medially and secured with wire fixation. Nasal augmentation is performed using a costochondral graft or previously resected bone from the T-shaped bone segment. Medial canthopexies are performed and secured to the reconstructed T-shaped bone or to the reconstructed nasal bone. Redundant soft tissue overlying the nose may be de-epithelialized and repurposed as a dermal flap if the overlying dorsal skin is too thin. Criticisms of the Chula technique center on the unaesthetic nasal incision, which does not adhere to principles of nasal subunits, the inability to correct the long nose deformity, and the preference to individually fixate the medial canthal tendons rather than en bloc repositioning with the bony medial orbit.

Orbital Hypertelorism

Medial orbital composite-unit translocation and HULA procedures
Boonvisut and colleagues[19] introduced the MOCUT in 2001 as an intracranial means to

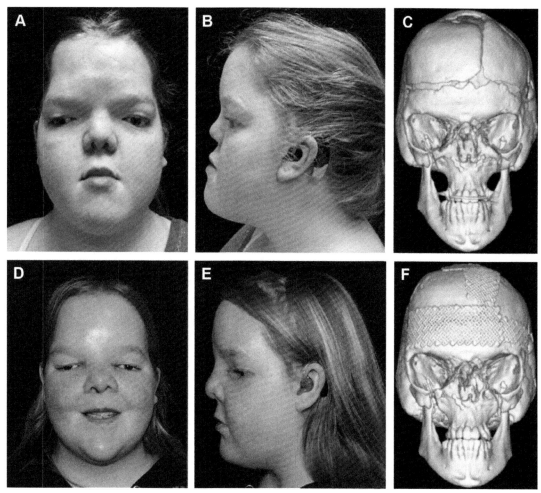

Fig. 2. (*A*) A 20-year-old woman with interorbital hypertelorism secondary to frontonasal dysplasia, anteroposterior view and (*B*) lateral view. (*C*) Preoperative CT scan. (*D*) Anteroposterior view and (*E*) lateral view 1.5 years after Le Fort II and Chula procedure. (*F*) Postoperative CT scan. The patient also underwent a titanium cranioplasty.

correct frontonasoethmoidal encephaloceles in interorbital hypertelorism (**Fig. 3**). This technique approaches the encephalocele through a small frontal craniotomy, in contrast to the extracranial approach popularized by Mahatumarat and colleagues.[18] The composite unit consists of the medial orbital rims, medial canthal ligaments, and lacrimal apparatus, which are subsequently transposed medially. Bone grafts taken from the resected bony excess and inner table of the craniotomy flap (or freeze-dried bone graft in children <3 months age) are then placed along the lateral aspects of the newly medialized composite unit along the superior orbital rim to reinforce the correction and to cover the internal bony defect, respectively. Compared with Mahatumarat's extracranial technique,[18] this technique obviates the need for alloplastic reconstruction of the

internal bony defect, improves exposure and subsequent repair of multiple internal bony defects (often observed in the series of Boonvisut and colleagues[19]), avoids unaesthetic nasal incisions, corrects telecanthus without transnasal medial canthopexies, and potentially avoids augmentation rhinoplasty by tilting the composite segment outward. Boonvisut and colleagues[19] argued that the ideal age of repair was approximately 3 months, as these children had considerably less interorbital distortion and bony telecanthus (ie, interorbital telecanthus).

In 2009, Kumar and colleagues[20] published their series of 12 patients undergoing an intracranial iteration similar to the MOCUT under the acronym HULA (H = hard-tissue sealant, U = undermine and excise encephalocele, L = lower supraorbital bar, A = augment nasal dorsum). The procedure

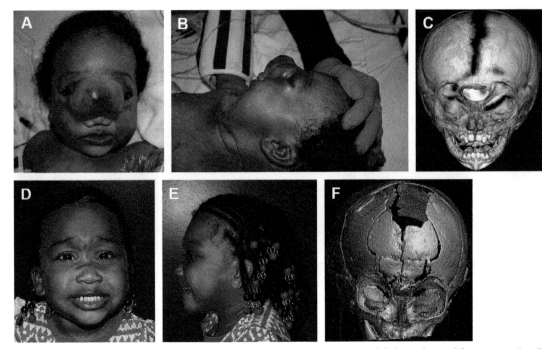

Fig. 3. A 3-month-old with frontonasal encephalocele, anteroposterior view (A), lateral view (B). Preoperative CT scan (C). Anteroposterior view (D) and lateral view (E) 1.5 years following MOCUT. Postoperative CT scan (F).

begins with an intracranial exposure through a limited frontal craniotomy and supraorbital bar excision to allow for ligation of the encephalocele stalk and subsequent dural repair. After transection of the encephalocele, the internal bony defect is sealed with split cranial bone graft, pericranial flaps, and fibrin glue. The second step involves undermining and dissecting the encephalocele mass either through an open approach directly over the nose (similar to the lambda-type incision popularized in the Chula technique) or through a closed approach using bilateral upper gingivobuccal sulcus incisions, intercartilaginous rhinoplasty incisions, and transconjunctival incisions for medial inferior orbital osteotomies. Bony reconstruction involves lowering the supraorbital bar, V-shape resection of the excess central bone, translocation of the medial orbital walls, and repositioning of the medial canthus using transnasal wires. Similar to the MOCUT technique, the resected accessory bone is used as graft material to reinforce the lateral aspects of the supraorbital bar. Nasal augmentation, a critical aspect of hypertelorism correction, used a separate full-thickness cranial bone graft superior to the frontal craniotomy as a cantilever nasal bone graft. The base of the graft is fixated at the level of the newly positioned medial canthi to replicate the low radix position inherent to the Southeast Asian ethnicity. Although the MOCUT and HULA procedures are

undeniably similar, the investigators reasoned that composite-unit medialization could not fully correct the superiorly displaced supraorbital region and anterolaterally displaced medial canthi. Consequently, the HULA procedure independently lowers the supraorbital bar while postero-medially translocating the medial canthal bone segment. The investigators also stress the importance of a low radix position for the augmented nasal dorsum using cantilever cranial bone graft, in comparison with the outward tilting of the composite segment in the MOCUT procedure.

Four-wall box osteotomy
Tessier reasoned that true orbital hypertelorism, unlike interorbital hypertelorism, must be corrected *intracranially*, as the inherent defect lies within the anterior cranial base (**Fig. 4**).[16,17] This concept deviated from the extracranial surgical techniques popularized by Webster and Deming,[7] Converse and colleagues,[8] and Schmid,[10] and ushered in an era of multidisciplinary craniofacial surgery by bridging the imaginary divide between the cranium and face. He introduced the 4-wall box osteotomy with the aim to "bring the eyes closer together by approximating the 'useful orbits,' without risking a meningeal infection or affecting ocular, oculomotor, or respiratory functions."[2] Hoffman and colleagues[21] later corroborated the importance of lateral wall medialization

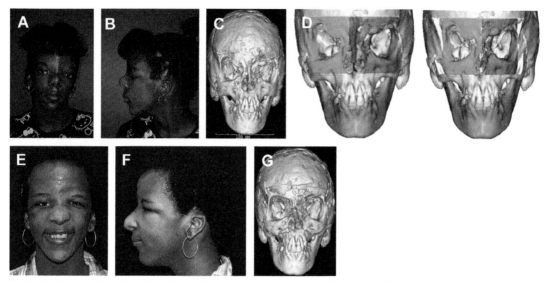

Fig. 4. A 12-year old with orbital hypertelorism secondary to craniofrontonasal dysplasia, anteroposterior view (*A*), lateral view (*B*). Preoperative CT scan (*C*). Virtual surgical plan for 4-wall box osteotomies (*D*). One year after 4-wall box osteotomies, anteroposterior view (*E*), lateral view (*F*). Postoperative CT scan (*G*).

in the correction of orbital hypertelorism through CT imaging analysis, a principle initially championed by Tessier during the late 1960s.[11]

Tessier's[2] original description of single-stage orbital hypertelorism correction outlined 13 key steps to guide true medialization of the bony orbits. First, a bicoronal skin flap is raised to allow for a frontal craniotomy with subsequent dura elevation off the anterior cranial base and to expose the malar bones and zygomatic arches distally. Dural tears are directly repaired or through use of pericranial flaps. Next, a midline incision over the nose allows for nasal and paranasal dissection from the underlying skeleton. The orbital floor and infraorbital region are then accessed through a transconjunctival approach, allowing for circumferential (ie, 4-wall) exposure and to within 10 mm of the optic foramen and supraorbital fissure posteriorly. Subsequent resection of accessory naso-fronto-ethmoidal tissue includes the floor of the anterior cranial base, frontal bone, ethmoid, nasal septum, and central processes of the maxillae. Intraorbital osteotomies and circumferential osteotomies of the orbital roof, lateral orbital wall, posteromedial wall, and orbital floor encompassing the infraorbital foramen then allow for en bloc medialization of the bony orbits and synchronous movement of nerves and vessels exiting the orbital apices. It should be noted that successful maxillary osteotomy requires adequate descent of the secondary teeth. After medial displacement of the orbits, the nasal mucosa and upper and lower lateral cartilages are repaired. Bone grafts are then placed laterally

along the medialized orbital roof, along the temporal fossa and zygoma gaps created by lateral osteotomies, and on the floor of the anterior cranial base. Medial canthopexies are performed using transnasal wiring in addition to nasal dorsal bone grafting. Last, the frontal craniotomy flap is fixated, the nasal soft tissues including the deformed cartilages are recontoured, and the incisions closed.

Several important factors and evolutions of the 4-wall or "box-shift" osteotomy must be considered. Tessier's[2] initial cases advocated for total ethmoidectomy and subsequent sacrifice of the olfactory nerves to comprehensively medialize the superomedial angles of the bony orbits. This medialization inherently led to olfaction obstruction, given its anatomic relation to the cribiform plate, which was often deformed. Interestingly, Tessier and colleagues[11] performed their first hypertelorism correction in 1962 as a 2-staged procedure: after olfactory sacrifice at the level of the cribiform plate, they interposed a dermal graft given concern for spread of infection into the subdural space. Converse and colleagues[8] are credited with the first successful intracranial olfaction-preserving (ie, cribiform-sparing) correction; a technique later adopted by Tessier in most of his cases. Tessier's[2] variation to the paramedian ethmoidectomy technique of Converse and colleagues[8] involved "anterior resections on each side of the nasal bridge" and preservation of a "keel"-shaped "narrow nasofrontal bridge." However, dissection and preservation of olfaction in relation to the cribiform plate remains a significant challenge given consistently aberrant anatomy and type and etiology of disease (ie, third-degree hypertelorism or the meningoencephalocele subtype) that may render the sense of olfaction inconsequential. An abnormally positioned (ie, too cephalad) cribiform plate and/or widely spaced olfactory grooves preclude paramedian resection of the ethmoidal cells and subsequent preservation of the olfactory nerves. Moreover, the crista galli may be enlarged, duplicated, or absent, in relation to various positions of the olfactory grooves.[2] Although dermal grafting to separate intracranial and intranasal contents is no longer indicated, dural repairs must be meticulous and reinforced with periosteal patches or pericranial flaps to prevent meningitis.

Importantly, the 4-wall box osteotomy allows for correction of symmetric and asymmetric deformities in all vectors (ie, vertical, horizontal, anterior, and posterior). Tessier's[2] original description details a "frontal crown" (ie, frontal bar) that not only provides stable bone-graft fixation of the newly repositioned orbits, but also safeguards against anterior malposition and subsequent postoperative enophthalmos. Moreover, the frontal crown serves as the proximal fixation point for the nasal dorsal bone graft. Marchac and Arnaud[22] recognized the importance of an anteroposterior landmark that provides a stable point of fixation, but argued that the frontal crown prevents ideal exposure of the anterior cranial base, as it lies at least 2 cm cephalad to the superior orbital rims. They consequently replaced Tessier's frontal crown with low lateral frontal spurs bilaterally created during frontal craniotomy that similarly provide stable fixation and precise repositioning without limiting the exposure to the anterior cranial base. This technical refinement allows for a more inferior positioned craniotomy with the caudal edge positioned 1 cm superior to the supraorbital rims. These lateral spurs begin at the level of the mid-orbit during creation of the frontal flap.

Tessier[2] highlighted the complexity in decision-making regarding hypertelorism correction. Although interorbital hypertelorism can generally be corrected through an extracranial approach, not all orbital hypertelorism warrants intracranial intervention. Fifty-two of Tessier's[2] initial 65 cases underwent intracranial orbital hypertelorism correction, which he advocated for in severe cases, pneumatized frontal bones, and orbital asymmetry. Contrastingly, he argued that caudal malposition of the cribiform plate precludes effective medialization via the intracranial approach given the mechanical barrier and risk of subdural infection. For Tessier,[2] the risks of intracranial surgery were unjustifiable in those patients affected by a mild form of orbital hypertelorism that may achieve similar results via an extracranial approach. In compiling his initial experience, Tessier[2] stated "the extracranial route should be used more often."

Facial bipartition

Van der Meulen[23] described the "medial fasciotomy" or facial bipartition in 1979 as an intracranial reconstructive technique aimed at simultaneous correction of orbital hypertelorism and midface deformity, specifically the V-shaped maxillary arch (**Fig. 5**). Instead of separating the orbit from the maxilla through an infraorbital osteotomy, van der Meulen performed a pterygomaxillary disjunction and midline division of the hard palate[21] to medialize the orbits, lengthen the midface, and correct the occlusion. Facial bipartition allows for (1) correction of orbital hypertelorism through a V-shaped bony wedge resection of the central face, (2) improved position of the displaced lateral canthi through orbital rotation, (3) correction of the "keel deformity" or V-shaped maxillary arch, (4) correction of the occlusal plane, and (5) preservation of the tooth buds. Medialization of each facial half occurs after midline V-shaped resection that is wider at the top, effectively reducing the interorbital distance and medially displacing the bony orbits. The triangular bony defects created at the superolateral aspects of the mobilized orbits are subsequently bone grafted. This V-shaped medial bony resection also corrects the "down and out" displacement and convexity of the lateral orbits and canthi after midline centralization to a more anatomic position.[22] Most importantly, pterygomaxillary disjunction and midline palatal split allows for correction of a transversely constricted, high-arched palate by lengthening and widening the midface, leveling the occlusal plane, and widening the nasal fossae. In contrast to the box osteotomy, there is no infraorbital cut to disrupt maxillary tooth buds in the growing craniofacial skeleton. Disadvantages to the bipartition include creation of a temporary gap between the maxillary central incisors and disruption of the pterygomaxillary buttresses. Marchac and Arnaud[22] used the bipartition procedure with and without LeFort III osteotomy in craniofrontonasal dysplasia cases (ie, Apert syndrome) as a second stage after traditional anterior or posterior skull expansion. It is our institutional practice to perform a facial bipartition when orbital hypertelorism also presents with a shortened midface or high-arched palate.

Soft Tissue Refinements

Tessier and colleagues[11] believed that hypertelorism correction "...has its real difficulties, not so

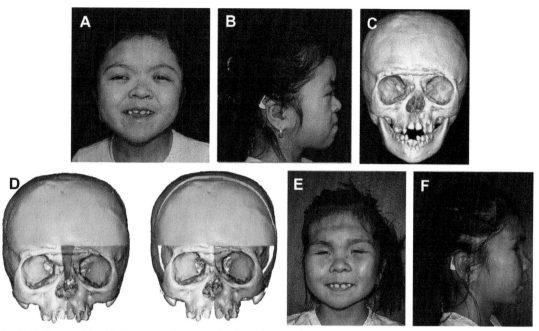

Fig. 5. A 9-year-old with Apert syndrome and orbital hypertelorism, anteroposterior view (*A*), lateral view (*B*). Preoperative CT scan (*C*). Virtual surgical plan for facial bipartition (*D*). Six months after facial bipartition, anteroposterior view (*E*), lateral view (*F*).

much in reducing an exaggerated interorbital distance as in correcting the other malformations which increase it or are associated with it." Contemporaries including John Converse and later Joseph McCarthy substantiated this claim by describing the difficulties in restoring the aesthetic "naso-orbital valley" and addressing the challenges beyond the "...bone carpentry...[namely] the nose and medial canthus."[24] We present 3 broad categories of soft tissue refinements based on the description of Raposo-Amaral and colleagues.[25]

Midline
The ideal timing and type of reconstruction to address midline soft tissue excess following bony hypertelorism correction remains to be determined.[26,27] Initial management included direct excision with primary closure at index operation, which results in a midline scar extending from the central forehead to the nasal tip.[7,8] The series of McCarthy and colleagues[28] suggested that excessive resection of midline soft tissues may lead to abnormal nasal development. Tessier[2] later proposed a Z-plasty at the frontonasal angle to medialize the eyebrows, while lengthening the nose, preventing epicanthal folds, and supporting canthopexies, similar to the figure-8 skin incision later popularized by Munro and Das.[29] To prevent an unpredictable amount of tissue resection during index operation and to avoid a midline scar,

Kawamoto and colleagues[27] more recently popularized the "K stitch," consisting of subcutaneous soft tissue excision in the medial region between the brows followed by multiple horizontal mattress sutures to optimize the brow position. The K stitch allows for revision direct excision, if needed, in a more predictable manner; however, the technique precludes the ability to perform total nasal reconstruction in severe cases using the paramedian forehead flap or scalping flap of Converse and McCarthy.[30]

Canthi and periorbita
The prevailing stigmata associated with hypertelorism correction relates to persistence of telecanthus, epicanthal folds, and loss of the "naso-orbital valley," a term coined by John Converse.[22] Soft tissue laxity in the medial canthal region leads to the illusion of bony relapse or inadequate correction, despite appropriately medialized bony orbits. Initial attempts at hypertelorism correction involved medial canthal detachment; however, this led to notable canthal drift in the postoperative period.[2] Postoperative medial canthal drift after canthus release led to the preference for canthus preservation during medial orbital wall osteotomy and transnasal wiring, which led to notable improvement.[31] Epicanthal folds may secondarily be addressed through Y-V plasty or double-opposing Z-plasty.[25,32]

Nasal

Tessier stated that "the correction of hypertelorism is surgery of the nose."[31] The importance of nasal augmentation cannot be understated, as midline forehead and glabellar scars can often be justified in the setting of an aesthetically pleasing reconstruction. Most (if not all) patients undergoing hypertelorism reconstruction require some form of secondary nasal reconstruction.[28,33] McCarthy[24] advocated for a sizable iliac corticocancellous nasal bone graft at time of index correction to not only augment the nose, but also to use midline soft tissue excess. Various grafting sites have been described, including cranial, rib, iliac, and midline bony excess at time of resection,[2,12,24,25] in addition to various surgical approaches (ie, open rhinoplasty, coronal incision). Tessier[2] advocated for the nasal bridge to be reconstructed with a rib bone graft bolted to the frontal bone and an auxiliary strut at the anterior nasal spine to support the graft. The bifid nose, a common presentation in patients with craniofrontonasal dysplasia, requires simultaneous bone grafting, nasal ala, and alar cartilage reshaping, namely the divergent medial crus. Raposo-Amaral and colleagues[25] advocate for primary midline soft tissue excision at index procedure in the setting of redundant soft tissue with adequately positioned nasal ala and alar cartilages. Paramedian forehead or scalping flap reconstruction combined with medialization of the divergent medial crura via interdomal suture technique can sufficiently correct more severe nasal phenotypes, in contrast. When performing the Converse scalping flap, the superficial temporal artery must be preserved, while the K stitch cannot be combined with paramedian forehead flap reconstruction to protect the vascular pedicles for total nasal reconstruction.

OUTCOMES

The most important outcome following bony correction of hypertelorism remains relapse and its relation to timing of surgery and future growth potential. Several conflicting reports exist within the literature. Early cephalometric studies completed by McCarthy and colleagues[28] and Lejoyeux and colleagues[34] suggested minimal bony relapse without hindering midfacial growth despite intervention at an early age (ie, younger than 5.3 years of age and 4–11 years of age, respectively). In his preliminary study, McCarthy and colleagues[28] noticed decreased maxillary growth in patients with cleft palate or facial clefts, inherently associated with maxillary hypoplasia, and impaired nasal development in patients undergoing excessive resection of midline soft tissue excess. Mulliken and colleagues[31] later published a series of 30 patients undergoing bony correction with mean age of 12 years and concluded that "early osteotomy across the upper maxilla in combination with nasoethmoidal resection may indeed interfere with anterior facial growth." They argued that relapse rates were higher in younger patients because of ongoing growth of the interorbital distance, and advocated for definitive bony correction in adolescence unless psychological reasons to intervene earlier presented themselves. Raposo-Amaral and colleagues[35] reviewed 22 patients during a 30-year period and concluded that relapse rates were significantly higher in patients undergoing correction when younger than 8 when compared with their older counterparts independent of severity and technique. In contrast, Marchac and colleagues[33] argued that age at time of correction was independent of future midfacial growth disturbance despite midline resection including the nasal septum. Nevertheless, there is unanimous agreement that the older patients achieve better and more lasting hypertelorism correction, given the cessation of craniofacial growth and thicker bones.

Complications

In the acute setting, bleeding, cerebrospinal fluid (CSF) leak, and infection remain the major postoperative complications associated with hypertelorism correction. CSF leak postoperatively may be treated either by repeat lumbar puncture or lumbar drain placement to prevent deadly complications of meningitis. Less common, but devastating, complications such as blindness and death have been reported, underscoring the invasive nature of transcranial procedures.[36,37] Late complications include the illusion of relapse due to soft tissue laxity in the medial canthal region, temporal hollowing amenable to fat grafting, and oculomotor disorders (ie, a preoperative exotropia that becomes an esotropia following bony correction).

REFERENCES

1. Demyer W, Zeman W, Palmer CG. The face predicts the brain: diagnostic significance of median facial anomalies for holoprosencephaly (arhinencephaly). Pediatrics 1964;34:256–63.
2. Tessier P. Experiences in the treatment of orbital hypertelorism. Plast Reconstr Surg 1974;53(1):1–18.
3. Greig DM. Hypertelorism: a hitherto undifferentiated congenital craniofacial deformity. Edinb Med J 1924; 31:560.

4. van der Meulen JC, Vaandrager JM. Surgery related to the correction of hypertelorism. Plast Reconstr Surg 1983;71(1):6–19.

5. Tan ST, Mulliken JB. Hypertelorism: nosologic analysis of 90 patients. Plast Reconstr Surg 1997;99(2):317–27.

6. van der Meulen J, Mazzola R, Stricker M, et al. Classification of craniofacial malformations. In: Stricker M, van der Meulen J, Raphael B, Mazzola R, editors. Craniofacial malformations. New York: Churchill-Livingstone; 1990.

7. Webster JP, Deming EG. The surgical treatment of the bifid nose. Plast Reconstr Surg (1946) 1950;6(1):1–37.

8. Converse JM, Ransohoff J, Mathews ES, et al. Ocular hypertelorism and pseudohypertelorism. Advances in surgical treatment. Plast Reconstr Surg 1970;45(1):1–13.

9. Troutman RC, et al. Plastic and reconstructive surgery of the eye and adnexa: Papers Presented to the First International Symposium of the Manhattan Eye, Ear and Throat Hospital. Butterworths. New York, 1962.

10. Schmid E. Surgical management of hypertelorism. In: Longacre JJ, editor. Craniofacial anomalies. Philadelphia: J. B. Lippincott Co.; 1968. p. 155.

11. Tessier P, Guiot G, Rougerie J, et al. Osteotomies cranio-naso-orbito-faciales hypertelorisme. Ann Chir Plast 1967;12:103.

12. Arnaud E, Marchac D, Di Rocco F, et al. Orbital hypertelorism. In: Rodriguez ED, Losee JE, Neligan PC, editors. Plastic surgery: craniofacial, head and neck surgery and pediatric plastic surgery, vol. 3. Elsevier Health Sciences; 2017. p. 685–700.

13. Tessier P. Anatomical classification facial, craniofacial and latero-facial clefts. J Maxillofac Surg 1976;4(2):69–92.

14. Mahatumarat C, Rojvachiranonda N, Taecholarn C. Frontoethmoidal encephalomeningocele: surgical correction by the Chula technique. Plast Reconstr Surg 2003;111(2):556–65 [discussion: 566–7].

15. Figalova P, Hajnis K, Smahel Z. The interocular distance in children with cleft before the operation. Acta Chir Plast 1974;16(2):65–77.

16. Tessier P. Orbital hypertelorism. I. Successive surgical attempts. Material and methods. Causes and mechanisms. Scand J Plast Reconstr Surg 1972;6(2):135–55.

17. Tessier P, Guiot G, Derome P. Orbital hypertelorism. II. Definite treatment of orbital hypertelorism (OR.H.) by craniofacial or by extracranial osteotomies. Scand J Plast Reconstr Surg 1973;7(1):39–58.

18. Mahatumarat C, Taecholarn C, Charoonsmith T. One-stage extracranial repair and reconstruction for frontoethmoidal encephalomeningocele: a new simple technique. J Craniofac Surg 1991;2(3):127–33 [discussion: 134].

19. Boonvisut S, Ladpli S, Sujatanond M, et al. A new technique for the repair and reconstruction of frontoethmoidal encephalomeningoceles by medial orbital composite-unit translocation. Br J Plast Surg 2001;54(2):93–101.

20. Kumar A, Helling E, Guenther D, et al. Correction of frontonasoethmoidal encephalocele: the HULA procedure. Plast Reconstr Surg 2009;123(2):661–9.

21. Hoffman WY, McCarthy JG, Cutting CB, et al. Computerized tomographic analysis of orbital hypertelorism repair: spatial relationship of the globe and the bony orbit. Ann Plast Surg 1990;25(2):124–31.

22. Marchac D, Arnaud E. Midface surgery from Tessier to distraction. Childs Nerv Syst 1999;15(11–12):681–94.

23. van der Meulen JC. Medial faciotomy. Br J Plast Surg 1979;32(4):339–42.

24. McCarthy JG. Discussion: hypertelorism correction: what happens with growth? Evaluation of a series of 95 surgical cases. Plast Reconstr Surg 2012;129(3):728–30.

25. Raposo-Amaral CE, Denadai R, Ghizoni E, et al. Surgical strategies for soft tissue management in hyperlorbitism. Ann Plast Surg 2017;78(4):421–7.

26. Caronni EP. Facial bipartition in hypertelorism. Cleft Palate J 1986;23(Suppl 1):19–26.

27. Urrego AF, Garri JI, O'Hara CM, et al. The K stitch for hyperlorbitism: improved soft tissue correction with glabellar width reduction. J Craniofac Surg 2005;16(5):855–9.

28. McCarthy JG, La Trenta GS, Breitbart AS, et al. Hypertelorism correction in the young child. Plast Reconstr Surg 1990;86(2):214–25 [discussion: 226–8].

29. Munro IR, Das SK. Improving results in orbital hypertelorism correction. Ann Plast Surg 1979;2(6):499–507.

30. Converse JM, McCarthy JG. The scalping forehead flap revisited. Clin Plast Surg 1981;8(3):413–34.

31. Mulliken JB, Kaban LB, Evans CA, et al. Facial skeletal changes following hyperorbitism correction. Plast Reconstr Surg 1986;77(1):7–16.

32. del Campo AF. Surgical treatment of the epicanthal fold. Plast Reconstr Surg 1984;73(4):566–71.

33. Marchac D, Sati S, Renier D, et al. Hypertelorism correction: what happens with growth? Evaluation of a series of 95 surgical cases. Plast Reconstr Surg 2012;129(3):713–27.

34. Lejoyeux E, Tulasne JF, Tessier PL. Maxillary growth following total septal resection in correction of orbital hypertelorism. Cleft Palate J 1986;23(Suppl 1):27–39.

35. Raposo-Amaral CE, Raposo-Amaral CM, Raposo-Amaral CA, et al. Age at surgery significantly impacts the amount of orbital relapse following hyperlorbitism correction: a 30-year longitudinal study. Plast Reconstr Surg 2011;127(4):1620–30.

36. Bradley JP, Gabbay JS, Taub PJ, et al. Monobloc advancement by distraction osteogenesis decreases morbidity and relapse. Plast Reconstr Surg 2006;118(7):1585–97.

37. Fearon JA, Whitaker LA. Complications with facial advancement: a comparison between the Le Fort III and monobloc advancements. Plast Reconstr Surg 1993;91(6):990–5.

Treacher Collins Syndrome

Albaraa Aljerian, MBBS[a], Mirko S. Gilardino, MD, MSc, FRCSC[b],*

KEYWORDS

- Treacher Collins syndrome • Franceschetti-Klein syndrome • Malar hypoplasia
- Mandibular hypoplasia • Mandibular distraction • Congenital airway • Facial deformity • Microtia

KEY POINTS

- Treacher Collins syndrome presents a challenge to the craniofacial plastic surgeon with both significant functional and aesthetic considerations.
- Recent data have elucidated the multilevel anatomic complexity of the airway in Treacher Collins syndrome. Mandibular distraction osteogenesis is an effective option in select patients; however, tracheostomy at times cannot be averted.
- Facial manifestations of the syndrome can produce significant psychosocial impact. Surgical treatment to obviate stigma are continually being developed and refined.
- Patients with Treacher Collins syndrome should be referred to specialized centers with the comprehensive care of a multidisciplinary craniofacial team.
- As a rare disorder, there remains a paucity of high-level evidence as to the treatment protocol of patients with Treacher Collins syndrome.

BACKGROUND

Treacher Collins syndrome (TCS) is a congenital craniofacial disorder characterized by malar and mandibulomaxillary hypoplasia and periorbital anomalies.[1] Although its eponymous name is credited to Edward Treacher Collins, a British ophthalmologist who described the condition in 1900, its original description was by Thomson in 1846 followed by Berry in 1889. Later in 1949, Franceschetti and Klein reviewed the disorder and proposed the term "mandibulofacial dysostosis" (Franceschetti-Klein syndrome).[2–5] To classify the disorder based on embryogenesis rather than the anatomically descriptive (facial cleft) classification of Tessier, Van der Meulen referred to the disorder as "zygotemporoauromandibular dysplasia," whereby associated malformations such as microtia, not explained by an underlying cleft, could be accounted for.[6,7]

As is the case with rare disorders, there remains a paucity of high-level evidence regarding the treatment strategies targeting TCS dysmorphology.[8] With that in mind, the treatment of patients affected with TCS follows the principles that guide craniofacial surgery with other such diagnoses—bony manipulation as a foundation followed by soft tissue reconstruction. Priority is given to functional issues followed by aesthetic concerns as patients progress to facial maturity. Owing to the complexity and wide array of anomalies, the management of children born with TCS benefits from a multidisciplinary team approach. In addition to the craniofacial plastic surgeon, the expertise of specialists in ophthalmology, ear, nose, and throat specialist, speech pathology, audiology, orthodontics, genetics, respirology, pediatrics, and intensive care may be necessary. Patient and family counseling is of key importance to arrive at a satisfactory quality of life, because these patients

Disclosure Statement: The authors have nothing to disclose.
[a] Division of Plastic and Reconstructive Surgery, McGill University Health Center, 1001 Decarie Boulevard, B05. 3310, Montreal, Quebec H4A 3J1, Canada; [b] H.B. Williams Craniofacial and Cleft Surgery Unit, Montreal Children's Hospital, Division of Plastic and Reconstructive Surgery, McGill University Health Center, 1001 Decarie Boulevard, B05.3310, Montreal, Quebec H4A 3J1, Canada
* Corresponding author.
E-mail address: mirko.gilardino@muhc.mcgill.ca

Clin Plastic Surg 46 (2019) 197–205
https://doi.org/10.1016/j.cps.2018.11.005

will likely require multiple interventions throughout childhood and often into adulthood.[9]

This review is not meant to be an exhaustive summary of the craniofacial surgical techniques that have remained largely unchanged, but instead to summarize general treatment concepts and to highlight areas of significant evolution. Perhaps the single most impressive advance has been in our understanding of the complexities of the airway in this population, opening the doors to a new era of surgical techniques to treat this difficult problem.

GENETICS AND PATHOGENESIS

TCS is an autosomal-dominant disorder with variable penetrance.[10] With no gender predilection, the incidence is estimated at 1 in 50,000 live births.[11,12] Mutations in the TCOF1, POLR1D, and POLR1C genes are complicit in the development of TCS, with the majority showing mutations in the TCOF1 locus on chromosome 5q31.3-q33.3 encoding for the *Treacle* protein, resulting in deficient ribosome biogenesis and subsequent neural crest cell insufficiency. A subset of patients with the disorder display no mutations.[10] Moreover, some studies report an autosomal-recessive pattern of inheritance (POLR1C).[13] Sixty percent of cases show spontaneous or de novo mutations and 40% have family-specific mutations. No phenotype/genotype correlation has been shown.[10]

Patients born with the disorder show broad variability in phenotypic presentation. Whereas some patients can display mild periorbital deformity that can be clinically subtle, others demonstrate a more complete phenotype with severe periorbital anomalies (downward slanting palpebral fissures, canthal dystopia, and colobomas),

maxillomandibular hypoplasia, and hairline displacement with variable forms of microtia (**Fig. 1**).[10] Notwithstanding the severity, the deformity is bilateral and generally symmetric. The main presenting features reflect that of the underlying malformation in structures developed from the first and second branchial arches.[1] Other malformations include microtia with associated conductive hearing loss and possible speech delay, mandibular hypoplasia, and retrognathia with possible airway sequelae and cleft palate (in 40% of cases).[14,15] Intellectual disability and other extrafacial anomalies (eg, cardiac malformations) have been reported in the context of the underlying genetic mutation.[10,16]

Genetic analysis remains the definitive method of diagnosis for TCS, either prenatally or postnatally.[17] The usefulness of prenatal ultrasound examination in the diagnosis of TCS has also been described. Despite having the ability to detect some of the characteristic facial features of TCS, ultrasound examination alone cannot differentiate between similar syndromes of facial dysostoses.[18–22] In addition, given that a subset of patients may have no genetic mutations, together with phenotypic variability and lack of phenotype–genotype correlation, the results of prenatal genetic testing must be interpreted cautiously.

AIRWAY AND MANDIBLE

Airway obstruction remains the main priority of management when present in this subset of patients. Pierre Robin sequence can be an underlying process in TCS airway compromise, resulting in obstructive sleep apnea or possibly life-threatening respiratory insufficiency.[8,23,24] In their cohort, Plomp and colleagues[25] found that 54%

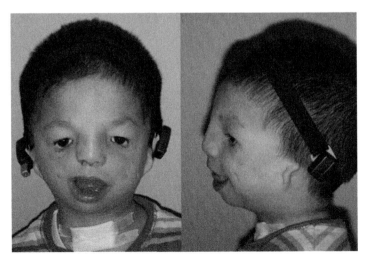

Fig. 1. Severe phenotype of Treacher Collins syndrome. (*Left*) periorbital malformations including downward slanting palpebral fissures and ectropion with scleral show. (*Right*) Microtia, low-lying ear remnants, and inferiorly displaced hairline. A band bone-anchored hearing aid is in place. (*From* Chang CC, Steinbacher DM. Treacher Collins syndrome. Semin Plast Surg 2012;26(2):84; with permission.)

of patients suffered from some form of obstructive sleep apnea, most being moderate, whereas Akre and colleagues[26] reported up to 95% of patients to be affected. Up to 78% of patients may display some form of mandibular involvement.[27,28] Any or all components of the mandible can be affected, including effacement of the mandibular angle, resulting in decreased posterior vertical height, a deep antegonial notch, and condylar aplasia with an aberrant temporomandibular joint.[29,30] Varying degrees of mandibular hypoplasia can be present.[31] When compared with hemifacial microsomia patients, the TCS mandibles as a whole were shown to be diminished volumetrically, exhibiting a volume comparable with Pruzansky type IIb and type III hemifacial microsomia mandibles.[32]

In severe cases, consultation with craniofacial surgeons will occur shortly after birth from the neonatal intensive care units. Focused evaluation typically begins with assessing positional oxygen saturation. Because the tongue proves to be relatively large in correlation to the oral cavity in the presence of micrognathia/retrognathia, desaturations are common in the supine position owing to aberrant oronasopharyngeal anatomy, glossoptosis, and airway obstruction.[33] Prone or decubitus positioning, as first-line management with or without a nasopharyngeal airway, can prove useful. If this is the case, outpatient management may be appropriate, because further growth of the mandible and airway will likely diminish the acute concern. If exogenous oxygen administration and/or positive airway pressure maneuvers are required, or if intubation is needed, further workup should be undertaken in the inpatient setting. Polysomnography, in addition to direct visualization methods such as laryngoscopy or bronchoscopy, are commonly used. These techniques help to delineate the cause of the apnea in question (central vs obstructive) and, more important, the level(s) of obstruction. In TCS, multiple anatomic airway anomalies are complicit in the obstructive pattern seen in certain patients.[23,34] Feeding difficulty should also be taken into account during patient assessment. Parenteral or enteral tube feeding methods may be required.

Surgical treatment, in the craniofacial context, is indicated if a compromised airway has been found to be due to a tongue-based obstruction or a diminished airway owing to retrognathia and mandibular hypoplasia, where the patient cannot be adequately managed by positioning or conservative measures alone.[35] Surgical procedures described include mandibular distraction osteogenesis, tongue–lip adhesion, and tracheostomy.[36–38] Genioplasty distraction osteogenesis with hyoid advancement has also been reported in patients who previously failed mandibular distraction.[39] The general goals of such surgical measures include decannulation or avoidance of tracheostomy and improvement of obstructive sleep apnea. Although correction of malocclusion and aesthetic differences (retrognathia) are sought, it is highly unlikely that such measures performed early in life for airway obstruction will persist into facial maturity and will likely have to be readdressed at a later stage.

Surgical planning includes preoperative imaging and direct airway assessment (flexible or rigid bronchoscopy) to rule out other airway anomalies that may be contributing to obstruction (including but not exclusive to laryngotracheomalacia, subglottic stenosis, vocal cord paralysis, septal deviation, choanal atresia, and hypertrophic adenoids).[33] Three-dimensional computed tomography imaging assists with the visualization of the anatomy and surgical planning (vectors of movement, osteotomy locations, etc), as well as an assessment of condylar or temporomandibular joint integrity.[30] Cephalometric radiographs can be useful in the context of assessing changes in craniofacial dimensions during and after treatment.

The TCS mandible should be addressed differently than patients with nonsyndromic Pierre Robin sequence, given the underlying morphology of the mandible.[40] The hypoplastic mandible in TCS can be deficient in 2 axes making the mandible uniplanar (**Fig. 2**).[41,42] In such cases, multivector distraction or curvilinear devices can be considered to address mandibular height and length in a single setting. Uniplanar devices, however, have also been demonstrated to have some usefulness in TCS cases in improving the 3-dimensional deficiency.[41] Regardless of technique, the timing of mandibular surgery remains debated. In cases where airway compromise is a factor, early distraction is an option to obviate the need for tracheostomy in select patients with adequate underlying anatomy. If airway is not a factor, then consideration can be given to delaying distraction or other facial osteotomies to maximize any native growth potential and decrease the need for repeat interventions owing to inevitable quantities of relapse, which can be significant or complete.

Recent studies have improved our understanding of the underlying complex airway anatomy in TCS patients that may predict the varying severity of the multifactorial airway obstruction. Ma and colleagues[23] have published 2 cross-sectional studies using 3-dimensional analyses to further clarify cephalometric changes in regard to cranial

	I	II	III	IV
SNB angle	Greater than 67°	62-67°	56-61°	Less than 55°
Co-Go-Me angle	Less than 135°	135-145°	146-155°	Greater than 155°
Condylar morphology	Normal	Morphologically normal, but hypoplastic/small	Condylar remnant that may not translate with glenoid fossa	Absent

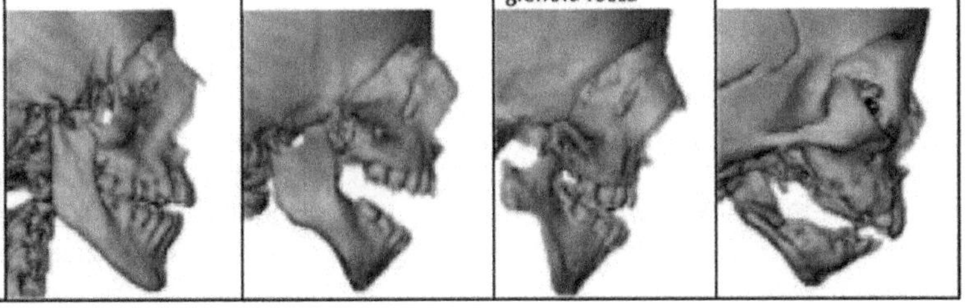

Fig. 2. Proposed classification of mandibular hypoplasia based on 3 categories: condylar morphology, retrognathia/sella–nasion–B point angle (SNB angle) and mandibular plane angle/Co-Go-Me angle. (*From* Ligh CA, Swanson J, Yu JW, et al, et al. A morphological classification scheme for the mandibular hypoplasia in Treacher Collins syndrome. J Craniofac Surg 2017;28(3):684; with permission.)

base, midface, and mandibular anomalous dimensions correlated with a smaller airway diameter.[34] Total upper airway volume was decreased by 30% with variability along its course; the most affected region being the retroglossal area. It was demonstrated that the length of the maxillary and mandibular bones, and anterior/posterior cranial base, were positively correlated with total airway volume. Alternatively, the mandibular projection (A-N-B angle) and the angle between the Frankfurt horizontal plane and mandible ramus plane (contributing to retrognathia) were negatively correlated. These results help to elucidate why mandibular distraction can (temporarily) improve airway patency. In a follow-up study by the authors focused on the nasal airway in this subset of patients, the nasal airway volume was found to be decreased by 40%. The most severely affected part is the anterior–inferior portion of the nasal cavity, demonstrating that transverse midface (ie, maxillary) hypoplasia, as well as its relative position or rotation, is a major factor.[23,34] Esenlik and colleagues[43] support this finding, reporting that retrognathia, decreased posterior facial height and an increase in the maxillary–mandibular plane angle were found to be correlated with the clinical severity of airway obstruction in the TCS population.

As mentioned elsewhere in this article, traditional techniques have focused on the surgical manipulation of the mandible alone. However, more recent airway data have delineated the contributory role of posterior facial height and the midfacial rotational deformity to the severity of airway obstruction.[29,44] To that end, recently a more innovative surgical approach has been described that addresses malposition of both the

midface and mandible. Hopper and colleagues[45] examined the effectiveness of counterclockwise craniofacial distraction osteogenesis (coined C3DO) to reestablish airway patency and successfully decannulate tracheostomy-dependent patients, some of whom failed previous mandibular distraction osteogenesis. In their cohort, 5 patients with tracheostomies underwent Lefort II, mandibular osteotomies and maxilla–mandibular fixation with subsequent rotation of the subcranial facial skeleton as a unit using external midface and mandibular distractors (**Fig. 3**). The authors demonstrated successful decannulation in 4 of 5 patients with a complex airway. Although in its infancy, this technique represents a significant step forward in our improved understanding and surgical management of the unique complexities of the TCS airway.

DENTITION AND PALATE

Cleft palate occurs with an estimated incidence of one-third of TCS patients.[14] There are no published data to suggest that timing of cleft repair should be any different than non-TCS patients. However, it has been reported that these patients can suffer from a higher incidence of fistula formation after repair, perhaps related to suboptimal vascular perfusion of the mucosa.[46,47] Special emphasis has been placed on speech and language rehabilitation, because the surgical results may be suboptimal owing to the underlying hypoplasia and tissue quality.[46] Anatomic differences can pose some difficulty at the time of repair, including decreased oral aperture and a high arched palate.[17]

Malocclusion is another common finding in TCS. An incidence of up to 94% of patients

A   **B**

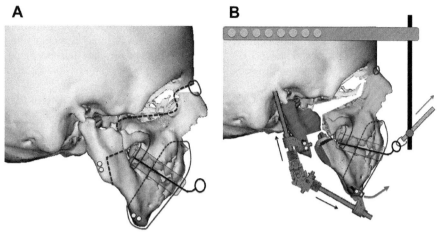

Fig. 3. Counterclockwise craniofacial distraction osteogenesis. (*A*) The Treacher Collins syndrome dysmorphology includes a clockwise rotation of the occlusal plane with associated airway deficit. (*B*) The subcranial skeleton is separated from the skull base through a Lefort II and bilateral mandibular osteotomies. A wire hinge is placed at the nasofrontal osteotomy and the patient is placed in maxillamandibular fixation. A midface distractor is attached to the maxillamandibular fixation splint and an external mandible distractor is placed with transfacial pins. The upward traction of the midface device creates a rotational force on the face and the mandible devices keep the mandibular condyle in position. Arrows: direction of pull. (*From* Hopper R, Kapadia H, Susarla S, et al. Counterclockwise craniofacial distraction osteogenesis (C3DO) for tracheostomy-dependent children with Treacher Collins syndrome. Plast Reconstr Surg 2018;142(2):449; with permission.)

demonstrating some form of malocclusion has been reported.[8] Typically, an anterior open bite with malpositioned teeth, often associated with a steep occlusal plane, is present.[17]

Some authors advocate the monitoring of dentition and oral hygiene as early as infancy, with subsequent orthodontic treatment once eruption of permanent teeth is complete.[48] Orthognathic intervention can take place during late adolescence. In the case of oral hygiene, one study concluded the presence of mild to severe salivary gland pathology in their cohort of 21 patients with TCS, resulting in oral dryness and higher prevalence of caries.[48]

PERIORBITAL FEATURES

Hypoplastic periorbital tissues are a hallmark of TCS (**Fig. 4**). The common finding of downward slanted palpebral (antimongoloid) fissures is related to lateral orbital wall hypoplasia/aplasia and the resultant canthal malposition.[17] Zygomaticomalar hypoplasia with a decrease in midfacial width and loss of normal protrusion of the cheeks is also common. Other periocular findings include colobomata of the lower eyelids and iris, ectropion, absence of eyelashes in the medial aspect of the lid, lacrimal system dysfunction or frank aplasia with resultant epiphora, strabismus, amblyopia, congenital cataracts, refractive errors, and/or vision loss.[17,49] The orbit is asymmetrically malformed, owing to the zygomatic hypoplasia.[50]

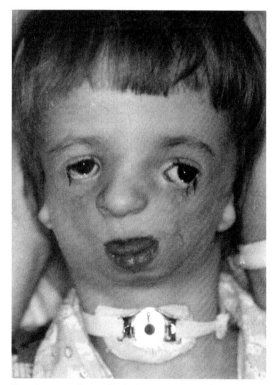

Fig. 4. A patient displaying a severe characteristic phenotype of Treacher Collins syndrome. Features include malar and mandibulomaxillary hypoplasia, periorbital soft tissue deficit with downward slanting palpebral fissures, lower lid colobomas, and ectropion. A tracheostomy is in place. (*From* Kobus K, Wojcicki P. Surgical treatment of Treacher Collins syndrome. Ann Plast Surg 2006;56(5):550; with permission.)

Surgical intervention is prioritized for procedures that minimize the risk of corneal desiccation and scarring (such as tarsorraphy), followed by those to address aesthetic deformities.[30] Techniques to correct lower lid abnormalities include Z-plasties, musculocutaneous advancement or transposition flaps (with or without prior tissue expansion) and canthopexy, among others.[28,51] Unfortunately, most described techniques are associated with visible scarring and contour deformities that are generally less than optimal.[1,27]

Zygomaticomalar hypoplasia is classically addressed with bone grafting, usually done in late childhood, with some authors advocating the procedures after the age of 7.[52] Fan and colleagues[52] have found a correlation between age of patient at time of grafting and degree of resorption, whereby as age increases, the likelihood of bony resorption decreases. Whereas costochondral grafts were used previously, newer data show a decreased rate of resorption when split or full-thickness calvarial bone grafts are used. McCarthy and colleague[53] has reported on the distraction of a bone graft used to augment the zygoma, obviating the need for repeat grafting, as is often required with this type of reconstruction given the degree of resorption and lack of growth potential. Another alternative is alloplastic reconstruction. Multiple reports have shown its usefulness, but it is not without risks commonly attributed to foreign material implantation, such as infection, malpositioning, migration, and extrusion.[54,55] Other techniques to correct midface hypoplasia that have been commonly described include Lefort I or II advancements to address the retropositioned maxilla.

Owing to the significant rates of resorption with nonvascularized bone grafting in the malar region, some authors have described the use of vascularized grafts, such as the temporal artery osteoperiosteal flap.[56] Despite its vascularized bony structure, the latter has been demonstrated to undergo significant resorption as well, limiting its popularity.[52]

In more recent years, fat grafting has increased in popularity owing to the minimal donor site morbidity and low-risk profile.[57] Harvest sites are similar to those in non-TCS patients; however, difficulty may arise in attempting to collect adequate amounts of adipose tissue, because these patients are commonly thin, with a slim body habitus.[8,58] Although requiring several sessions, fat grafting has proven to provide excellent malar volume augmentation, with early fat grafting advocated.[57]

Saadeh and colleagues[59] have reported on the use of free tissue transfer for the reconstruction of midface dysmorphology in patients with TCS, commonly from tissue harvested off the scapular system. Although effective in transporting significant volume to the face in a single setting, these patients required routine flap revisions to correct issues, such as sagging or volume asymmetry.

EAR MALFORMATION AND HEARING

Ear involvement is another common finding in TCS, with an incidence of anomalies reported up to 87%. Ears can show varying degrees of microtia, or in some cases, anotia. The position of the ears as well as the hairline can be low lying (in up to 48% of patients) (**Fig. 5**).[10] The external auricular deformity is commonly associated with a stenotic or atretic external auditory meatus and a malformed or absent middle ear.[17]

Up to 96% of patients are reported to have some degree of hearing loss.[10] A correlation between the severity of external auditory canal malformation and hearing impairment has been shown.[1] As a corollary, speech impairment may be present owing either to uncorrected hearing loss or other factors such maladaptive oral development.[60] In any case, an assessment by an ear, nose, and throat specialist, audiologist, and speech and language pathologist is essential.[46]

With regard to ear reconstruction, autologous methods have been advocated by most investigators, with the most commonly used techniques being those described by Nagata or Brent.[61,62]

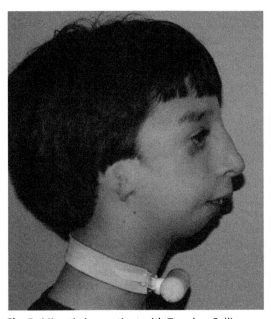

Fig. 5. Microtia in a patient with Treacher Collins syndrome. Low-lying ears and inferiorly displaced hairline are characteristic. (*From* Chang CC, Steinbacher DM. Treacher Collins syndrome. Semin Plast Surg 2012;26(2):85; with permission.)

Although autologous reconstruction remains as the most common technique, the use of porous polyethylene implants have also been described.[63] There is no evidence that the timing of surgery or the technique used should be any different with TCS patients as compared with other cohorts with microtia; however, the reconstruction of surrounding tissue, and the timing thereof, should be taken into account. Owing to the low-lying hairline characteristic of this subset of patients, laser hair removal has been advocated to ameliorate this concern.[10] The status of the superficial temporal artery affects decisions made for free tissue transfer.[64] Previous mandibular interventions should be noted, because this might affect the periauricular skin that is eventually included in microtia repair.[59,65] In addition, multidisciplinary planning is required to incorporate the ideal timing and location of bone-anchored hearing aid insertion if indicated as these 2 procedures may occupy similar anatomic real estate, causing some to place the fixture at a greater distance than usual from the meatus.[66] Another issue that can be faced is the insufficiency of calvarial bone thickness present in TCS patients that is not frequent in their nonsyndromic counterparts.[66]

Hearing impairment is typically addressed with removable bone-anchored hearing aid bands before definitive ear reconstruction.[30,66] This serves to prevent delay in language development, pending physical maturity to allow for definitive, commonly staged, ear reconstruction before conclusive osseointegrated bone-anchored hearing aid placement.[30]

SUMMARY

TCS is a complex multifaceted disorder that affects form and function. Patients suffering from the disorder should be referred to specialized centers that use a multidisciplinary team approach. Standard craniofacial techniques are the mainstay of current treatment protocols, although the type, timing, and role of mandibular surgery (distraction) continues to evolve. In addition, a more recent appreciation of the panfacial airway anomalies that contribute to the airway obstruction and aesthetic deformity will likely produce more stable and profound surgical correction of these anatomic issues. To that end, further research is still required to establish a more unified approach to this population.

REFERENCES

1. Posnick JC, Tiwana PS, Costello BJ. Treacher Collins syndrome: comprehensive evaluation and treatment. Oral Maxillofac Surg Clin North Am 2004;16(4):503–23.
2. Berry G. Note on a congenital defect (coloboma?) of the lower lid. R Lond Ophthalmol Hosp Rep 1889;12: 255–7.
3. Collins E. Cases of symmetrical congenital notches in the outer part of each lower lid and defective development of the malar bones. Trans Ophthalmol Soc U K 1900;20:190–2.
4. Franceschetti AKD. The mandibulofacial dysostosis; a new hereditary syndrome. Acta Ophthalmol (Copenh) 1949;27:143–224.
5. Thomson A. Notice of several cases of malformation of the external ear, together with experiments on the state of hearing in such persons. Mont J Med Sci 1846;7:420.
6. van der Meulen JC, Mazzola R, Vermey-Keers C, et al. A morphogenetic classification of craniofacial malformations. Plast Reconstr Surg 1983;71(4):560–72.
7. Tessier P. Anatomical classification facial, craniofacial and latero-facial clefts. J Maxillofac Surg 1976;4(2):69–92.
8. Plomp RG, van Lieshout MJ, Joosten KF, et al. Treacher Collins syndrome: a systematic review of evidence-based treatment and recommendations. Plast Reconstr Surg 2016;137(1):191–204.
9. de Oliveira JP, Lodovichi FF, Gomes MB, et al. Patient-reported quality of life in the highest functioning patients with Treacher Collins syndrome. J Craniofac Surg 2018;29(6):1430–3.
10. Vincent M, Genevieve D, Ostertag A, et al. Treacher Collins syndrome: a clinical and molecular study based on a large series of patients. Genet Med 2016;18(1):49–56.
11. Rovin S, Dachi SF, Borenstein DB, et al. Mandibulofacial dysostosis, a familial study of five generations. J Pediatr 1964;65:215–21.
12. Cunningham ML. Syndromes of the head and neck, Fourth Edition, by RJ Gorlin, MM Cohen, and RCM. Hennekam. Am J Med Genet 2002;113(3):312.
13. Dauwerse JG, Dixon J, Seland S, et al. Mutations in genes encoding subunits of RNA polymerases I and III cause Treacher Collins syndrome. Nat Genet 2011;43(1):20–2.
14. Peterson-Falzone S, Pruzansky S. Cleft palate and congenital palatopharyngeal incompetency in mandibulofacial dysostosis: frequency and problems in treatment. Cleft Palate J 1976;13:354–60.
15. Teber OA, Gillessen-Kaesbach G, Fischer S, et al. Genotyping in 46 patients with tentative diagnosis of Treacher Collins syndrome revealed unexpected phenotypic variation. Eur J Hum Genet 2004; 12(11):879–90.
16. Vincent M, Collet C, Verloes A, et al. Large deletions encompassing the TCOF1 and CAMK2A genes are responsible for Treacher Collins syndrome with intellectual disability. Eur J Hum Genet 2014;22(1):52–6.

17. Trainor PA, Dixon J, Dixon MJ. Treacher Collins syndrome: etiology, pathogenesis and prevention. Eur J Hum Genet 2008;17:275.

18. Cohen J, Ghezzi F, Goncalves L, et al. Prenatal sonographic diagnosis of Treacher Collins syndrome: a case and review of the literature. Am J Perinatol 1995;12(6):416–9.

19. Hsu TY, Hsu JJ, Chang SY, et al. Prenatal three-dimensional sonographic images associated with Treacher Collins syndrome. Ultrasound Obstet Gynecol 2002;19(4):413–22.

20. Meizner I, Carmi R, Katz M. Prenatal ultrasonic diagnosis of mandibulofacial dysostosis (Treacher Collins syndrome). J Clin Ultrasound 1991;19(2):124–7.

21. Ochi H, Matsubara K, Ito M, et al. Prenatal sonographic diagnosis of Treacher Collins syndrome. Obstet Gynecol 1998;91(5 Pt 2):862.

22. Tanaka Y, Kanenishi K, Tanaka H, et al. Antenatal three-dimensional sonographic features of Treacher Collins syndrome. Ultrasound Obstet Gynecol 2002; 19(4):414–5.

23. Ma X, Forte AJ, Persing JA, et al. Reduced three-dimensional airway volume is a function of skeletal dysmorphology in Treacher Collins syndrome. Plast Reconstr Surg 2015;135(2):382e–92e.

24. Evans KN, Sie KC, Hopper RA, et al. Robin sequence: from diagnosis to development of an effective management plan. Pediatrics 2011; 127(5):936–48.

25. Plomp RG, Bredero-Boelhouwer HH, Joosten KF, et al. Obstructive sleep apnoea in Treacher Collins syndrome: prevalence, severity and cause. Int J Oral Maxillofac Surg 2012;41(6): 696–701.

26. Akre H, Overland B, Asten P, et al. Obstructive sleep apnea in Treacher Collins syndrome. Eur Arch Otorhinolaryngol 2012;269(1):331–7.

27. Plomp RG, Versnel SL, van Lieshout MJ, et al. Long-term assessment of facial features and functions needing more attention in treatment of Treacher Collins syndrome. J Plast Reconstr Aesthet Surg 2013;66(8):e217–26.

28. Kobus K, Wojcicki P. Surgical treatment of Treacher Collins syndrome. Ann Plast Surg 2006;56(5): 549–54.

29. Chong DK, Murray DJ, Britto JA, et al. A cephalometric analysis of maxillary and mandibular parameters in Treacher Collins syndrome. Plast Reconstr Surg 2008;121(3):77e–84e.

30. Chang CC, Steinbacher DM. Treacher Collins syndrome. Semin Plast Surg 2012;26(2):83–90.

31. Ligh CA, Swanson J, Yu JW, et al. A morphological classification scheme for the mandibular hypoplasia in Treacher Collins syndrome. J Craniofac Surg 2017;28(3):683–7.

32. Travieso R, Terner J, Chang C, et al. Mandibular volumetric comparison of Treacher Collins syndrome and hemifacial microsomia. Plast Reconstr Surg 2012;129(4):749e–51e.

33. Biskup NI, Pan BS, Elhadi-Babiker H, et al. Decannulation and airway outcomes with maxillomandibular distraction in Treacher Collins and Nager syndrome. J Craniofac Surg 2018;29(3):692–7.

34. Ma X, Forte AJ, Berlin NL, et al. Reduced three-dimensional nasal airway volume in Treacher Collins syndrome and its association with craniofacial morphology. Plast Reconstr Surg 2015;135(5): 885e–94e.

35. Thompson JT, Anderson PJ, David DJ. Treacher Collins syndrome: protocol management from birth to maturity. J Craniofac Surg 2009;20(6): 2028–35.

36. Sculerati N, Gottlieb MD, Zimbler MS, et al. Airway management in children with major craniofacial anomalies. Laryngoscope 1998;108(12):1806–12.

37. Anderson PJ, Netherway DJ, Abbott A, et al. Mandibular lengthening by distraction for airway obstruction in Treacher-Collins syndrome: the long-term results. J Craniofac Surg 2004;15(1):47–50.

38. Argamaso RV. Glossopexy for upper airway obstruction in Robin sequence. Cleft Palate Craniofac J 1992;29(3):232–8.

39. Heller JB, Gabbay JS, Kwan D, et al. Genioplasty distraction osteogenesis and hyoid advancement for correction of upper airway obstruction in patients with Treacher Collins and Nager syndromes. Plast Reconstr Surg 2006;117(7):2389–98.

40. Chung MT, Levi B, Hyun JS, et al. Pierre Robin sequence and Treacher Collins hypoplastic mandible comparison using three-dimensional morphometric analysis. J Craniofac Surg 2012;23(7 Suppl 1):1959–63.

41. Singh DJ, Glick PH, Bartlett SP. Mandibular deformities: single-vector distraction techniques for a multivector problem. J Craniofac Surg 2009;20(5): 1468–72.

42. Stelnicki EJ, Lin WY, Lee C, et al. Long-term outcome study of bilateral mandibular distraction: a comparison of Treacher Collins and Nager syndromes to other types of micrognathia. Plast Reconstr Surg 2002;109(6):1819–25 [discussion: 1826–17].

43. Esenlik E, Plana NM, Grayson BH, et al. Cephalometric predictors of clinical severity in Treacher Collins syndrome. Plast Reconstr Surg 2017; 140(6):1240–9.

44. Arvystas M, Shprintzen RJ. Craniofacial morphology in Treacher Collins syndrome. Cleft Palate Craniofac J 1991;28(2):226–30 [discussion: 230–1].

45. Hopper R, Kapadia H, Susarla S, et al. Counterclockwise craniofacial distraction osteogenesis (C3DO) for tracheostomy-dependent children with Treacher Collins syndrome. Plast Reconstr Surg 2018;142(2):447–57.

46. Golinko MS, LeBlanc EM, Hallett AM, et al. Long-term surgical and speech outcomes following palatoplasty in patients with Treacher-Collins syndrome. J Craniofac Surg 2016;27(6):1408–11.
47. Bresnick S, Walker J, Clarke-Sheehan N, et al. Increased fistula risk following palatoplasty in Treacher Collins syndrome. Cleft Palate Craniofac J 2003;40(3):280–3.
48. da Silva Dalben G, Teixeira das Neves L, Ribeiro Gomide M. Oral health status of children with Treacher Collins syndrome. Spec Care Dentist 2006;26(2):71–5 [quiz: 85–77].
49. Hertle RW, Ziylan S, Katowitz JA. Ophthalmic features and visual prognosis in the Treacher-Collins syndrome. Br J Ophthalmol 1993;77(10):642–5.
50. Levasseur J, Nysjo J, Sandy R, et al. Orbital volume and shape in Treacher Collins syndrome. J Craniomaxillofac Surg 2018;46(2):305–11.
51. Ueda K, Nuri T, Shigemura Y. Malar reconstruction using Y-V advancement flaps after tissue expansion in Treacher Collins syndrome. Plast Reconstr Surg Glob Open 2016;4(5):e715.
52. Fan KL, Federico C, Kawamoto HK, et al. Optimizing the timing and technique of Treacher Collins orbital malar reconstruction. J Craniofac Surg 2012;23(7 Suppl 1):2033–7.
53. McCarthy JG, Hopper RA. Distraction osteogenesis of zygomatic bone grafts in a patient with Treacher collins syndrome: a case report. J Craniofac Surg 2002;13(2):279–83.
54. Roddi R, Vaandrager JM, van der Meulen JC. Treacher Collins syndrome: early surgical treatment of orbitomalar malformations. J Craniofac Surg 1995;6(3):211–7.
55. Sainsbury DC, George A, Forrest CR, et al. Bilateral malar reconstruction using patient-specific polyether ether ketone implants in Treacher-Collins syndrome patients with absent zygomas. J Craniofac Surg 2017;28(2):515–7.
56. van der Meulen JC, Hauben DJ, Vaandrager JM, et al. The use of a temporal osteoperiosteal flap for the reconstruction of malar hypoplasia in Treacher Collins syndrome. Plast Reconstr Surg 1984;74(5): 687–93.
57. Konofaos P, Arnaud E. Early fat grafting for augmentation of orbitozygomatic region in Treacher Collins syndrome. J Craniofac Surg 2015;26(4):1258–60.
58. Lim AA, Fan K, Allam KA, et al. Autologous fat transplantation in the craniofacial patient: the UCLA experience. J Craniofac Surg 2012;23(4):1061–6.
59. Saadeh P, Reavey PL, Siebert JW. A soft-tissue approach to midfacial hypoplasia associated with Treacher Collins syndrome. Ann Plast Surg 2006; 56(5):522–5.
60. Vallino-Napoli LD. A profile of the features and speech in patients with mandibulofacial dysostosis. Cleft Palate Craniofac J 2002;39(6):623–34.
61. Brent B. Microtia repair with rib cartilage grafts: a review of personal experience with 1000 cases. Clin Plast Surg 2002;29(2):257–71, vii.
62. Nagata S. Total auricular reconstruction with a three-dimensional costal cartilage framework. Ann Chir Plast Esthet 1995;40(4):371–99 [discussion: 400–3].
63. Reinisch JF, Lewin S. Ear reconstruction using a porous polyethylene framework and temporoparietal fascia flap. Facial Plast Surg 2009;25(3):181–9.
64. Maeda T, Oyama A, Funayama E, et al. Reconstruction of low hairline microtia of Treacher Collins syndrome with a hinged mastoid fascial flap. Int J Oral Maxillofac Surg 2016;45(6):731–4.
65. Kurabayashi T, Asato H, Suzuki Y, et al. A temporoparietal fascia pocket method in elevation of reconstructed auricle for microtia. Plast Reconstr Surg 2017;139(4):935–45.
66. Marsella P, Scorpecci A, Pacifico C, et al. Bone-anchored hearing aid (BAHA) in patients with Treacher Collins syndrome: tips and pitfalls. Int J Pediatr Otorhinolaryngol 2011;75(10):1308–12.

Craniofacial Microsomia

Craig Birgfeld, MD[a],*, Carrie Heike, MD, MS[b]

KEYWORDS

- Craniofacial microsomia • Hemifacial microsomia • Goldenhar syndrome
- Oculoauriculovertebral syndrome • Virtual surgical planning • Orthognathic surgery
- Distraction osteogenesis • Phenotypic assessment tool – craniofacial microsomia (PAT-CFM)

KEY POINTS

- Patients with craniofacial microsomia display a wide spectrum of phenotypic severity.
- Multiple clinical classification systems exist for the facial features in craniofacial microsomia.
- Treatment algorithms should be individualized for the patient's phenotype, functional needs, and preferences.
- Further research is required to evaluate optimal timing and type of treatments.
- The patients' complex needs are best treated by a multidisciplinary craniofacial team.

INTRODUCTION

Clinicians use different diagnostic terms for patients with underdevelopment of facial features arising from the embryonic first and second pharyngeal arches,[1–4] including first and second branchial arch syndrome, otomandibular dysostosis, oculoauriculovertebral syndrome,[5] and hemifacial microsomia. Recently, craniofacial microsomia (CFM) has been the preferred term, and encompasses the wide variety of phenotypic presentation. Although no diagnostic criteria for CFM exist, most patients have a degree of underdevelopment of the mandible, maxilla, ear, orbit, facial soft tissue, and/or facial nerve. These anomalies can affect feeding, compromise the airway, alter facial movement, disrupt hearing, and alter facial appearance. Children with CFM are best cared for by a multidisciplinary team. In fact, CFM occurs in as many as 1:3000 to 1:5000 live births[6,7] and it is the second most common congenital disorder of the face treated by craniofacial teams.[1,3]

PATHOGENESIS

The first and second pharyngeal arches form around the fourth week of embryologic development and give rise to the structures of the face innervated by cranial nerves V and VII. The first branchial arch gives rise to the maxilla, mandible, zygoma, trigeminal nerve, muscles of mastication, and the anterior portion of the ear (tragus, root, and superior helix) as well as the malleolus and incus. The second branchial arch gives rise to the hyoid bone, the styloid process and facial nerve, the facial muscles and most of the ear (helix, antihelix, antitragus, and lobule), as well as the stapes. For these structures to fully form, the mesenchymal cells of the arches must maintain continuous tissue-to-tissue communication to support the development of the skeletal, muscular, and neural components.[8–10] Disruption of this communication can result in hypoplasia or aplasia of the affected structure.[11]

CFM may result from disruption of this cellular communication by vascular injury, teratogen exposure, or genetic causes. Poswillo[12] conducted a series of experiments in which he caused a hematoma of the stapedial artery in mice by administering a teratogen (trazine) in the sixth week of gestation. Affected mice exhibited facial features similar to those seen in CFM. The stapedial artery supplies blood to the first and second

The authors have nothing to disclose.
[a] Pediatric Plastic and Craniofacial Surgery, Seattle Children's Hospital, 4800 Sand Point Way, M/S OB.9.520, PO Box 5371, Seattle, WA 98105, USA; [b] Craniofacial Pediatrics, Seattle Children's Hospital, 4800 Sand Point Way, M/S OB.9.528, PO Box 5371, Seattle, WA 98105, USA
* Corresponding author.
E-mail address: craig.birgfeld@seattlechildrens.org

Clin Plastic Surg 46 (2019) 207–221
https://doi.org/10.1016/j.cps.2018.12.001

pharyngeal arches, and the authors concluded that a vascular insult to the developing arches could be the cause of CFM, and that the phenotypic variation in CFM may reflect the degree of vascular disruption. Recent studies have identified associations with other maternal risk factors, such as the use of vasoactive medications, smoking during the second trimester, diabetes, and the use of reproductive technology.[13,14] Additional evidence exists for a genetic cause.[15–18] Inheritance patterns consistent with autosomal dominance with incomplete penetrance have been described in families[19–22] and, in a large series of cases, 50% had a positive family history.[23,24] Several chromosomal abnormalities have been detected in CFM.[25–30] Etiologic heterogeneity combined with incomplete penetrance and variable expression may account for the diverse phenotypic spectrum observed in CFM.

PRESENTATION AND DIFFERENTIAL DIAGNOSIS

Most physicians agree that the diagnosis of CFM requires the underdevelopment of 1 or more of the facial structures emanating from the first and second branchial arches; however, no established diagnostic criteria exist. Should patients with isolated microtia be included in the CFM spectrum? How should we classify patients with isolated macrostomia? Do patients with bilateral branchial remnants and no other facial features have CFM? A lack of consensus on the diagnostic criteria greatly impacts our ability to study the prevalence and critically evaluate existing treatment protocols. When comparing the SAT and OMENS systems, Cousley[31] recommended the following minimal diagnostic criteria:

1. Ipsilateral mandibular and ear defects.
2. Asymmetrical mandibular or ear defects in association with:
   a. Two or more indirectly associated anomalies, and
   b. A positive family history of CFM.

Anomalies such as microtia and mandibular hypoplasia are associated with many established syndromes with overlapping features of CFM. It is important to evaluate for features of CHARGE (coloboma, heart defect, atresia choanae [also known as choanal atresia], restricted growth and development, genital abnormality, and ear abnormality), Treacher–Collins, Nager, and other syndromes, given that these diagnoses will greatly influence treatment recommendations.

Patients with CFM present with signs and symptoms that result from their phenotype. Neonates with severe micrognathia often present with upper airway obstruction and failure to thrive. In this instance, the mandibular hypoplasia associated with CFM, which is often asymmetric, should be distinguished from the hypoplasia observed in Robin sequence (RS).[32] There is growth potential in RS[32] and treatments such as prone positioning, nasopharyngeal airways, and tongue lip adhesions may serve as effective temporizing measures in early infancy.[33] However, these interventions are not typically effective in infants with CFM, because the mandible does not display catch up growth and studies have not demonstrated that neonatal distraction osteogenesis is effective in children with CFM.

CLASSIFICATION

The initial phenotypic classifications schemes in CFM focused on the mandible. The Pruzansky classification system[34] organized the underdeveloped mandible into 3 groups (**Table 1**) based on radiographic features. Kaban and associates[35,36] later modified this system to describe the position of the temporomandibular joint (TMJ; **Table 2**). In this system, the IIA mandible displays a short ramus, but the glenoid fossa is in a normal position, whereas the IIB mandible has a malpositioned glenoid fossa that is typically anterior. They felt that the IIB mandible required reconstruction of the TMJ whereas the IIA mandible did not. This classification system, as well as others that incorporate 3-dimensional mandible images,[37–40] are widely used, and can be helpful guides to treatment of the mandibular deformity in CFM.

Other classification systems have been created to better describe the phenotype of all components of the face.[41–44] The SAT system, created by David and colleagues,[45] described the severity of skeletal, auricle, and soft tissue features in CFM, and is based on the approach used in the TNM classification system for tumors. Recommendations for surgical interventions are based on severity of SAT scores.

Table 1 Pruzansky classification 1969	
Grade	Characteristics
I	Smaller than preserved normal side
II	Condyle, ramus, and sigmoid notch identifiable, but grossly distorted in size and shape
III	Grossly distorted ramus with loss of landmarks or agenesis

From Pruzansky S. Not all dwarfed mandibles are alike. Birth Defects 1969;1:120–9; with permission.

Table 2
Kaban modification of the Pruzansky classification

Grade	Characteristics
I	Small mandible
IIA	Short mandibular ramus of abnormal shape; glenoid fossa in satisfactory position
IIB	Temporomandibular joint abnormally placed inferiorly, medially and anteriorly
III	Absent temporomandibular joint

From Kaban LB, Moses MH, Mulliken JB. Surgical correction of hemifacial microsomia in the growing child. Plast Reconstr Surg 1988;82:9–19; with permission

The most inclusive[31] and likely the most widely used, classification system is Vento's O.M.E.N.S.,[46] later modified to O.M.E.N.S+ to include extracranial mainfestations.[47] The acronym stands for orbit, mandible, ear, nerve, soft tissue, and each component is assigned a score from 0 to 3 based on severity. A pictorial representation was created[48] and modified to the PAT-CFM[49] to improve ease of use. The purpose of these classification systems is to create a shared vocabulary to describe complex phenotypic variation in patients with CFM to facilitate communication, evaluation of treatments and research.[50]

EVALUATION AND TREATMENT

Evaluations and interventions should be timed with craniofacial growth and tailored to the individual based on clinical characteristics and patient preferences. We include our previously published timeline as a general guide for practitioners and patients to consider options and timing of evaluations and treatments (**Fig. 1**).

General screening recommendations include audiologic evaluation to identify the presence and degree of hearing loss, along with cervical spine films and a renal ultrasound examination to detect common extracranial manifestations associated with CFM. Iterative, multidisciplinary assessments should continue throughout childhood for developmental surveillance[51] and assessment of psychosocial[52,53] health, hearing status, speech, and other common health considerations.

Additional evaluations are based on individual needs. For example, infants with CFM may demonstrate failure to thrive owing to symptoms of obstructive sleep apnea. In a multicenter study of 755 individuals with CFM, obstructive sleep apnea was identified in 17.6% of patients as compared with 2% to 4% of the general population and was correlated with worsening Pruzansky score.[54] In the same cohort, 13.5% of patients displayed oral and pharyngeal swallowing difficulty that correlated with increasing severity of Pruzansky classification.[55] The authors attributed this difficulty to functional or structural deficits in the pharynx, larynx, or esophagus[56]; mandibular hypoplasia; and/or decreased innervation of the masticatory and pharyngeal muscles.[57–59] Additionally, the presence of a cleft lip and/or palate (present in 15.9% of patients with CFM)[60] and abnormalities in the tongue[61–63] could contribute to feeding challenges. Therefore, additional evaluations for individuals with CFM often include an airway evaluation and/or polysomnography and, in patients with micrognathia and obstructive sleep symptoms, feeding evaluations in those at risk for dysphagia.

In addition to airway and feeding challenges, a large percentage of patients with CFM (35%) demonstrate extracranial involvement, and the likelihood increases in those with more severe phenotypes and with bilateral facial involvement.[64] Historically, patients with CFM, epibulbar dermoids, and vertebral anomalies were considered to have Goldenhar syndrome[65] (**Fig. 2**). Yet, the extracranial findings are not limited to this classic triad,[47] and many clinicians have recommended discontinuing the use of this term.[64,66,67]

SURGICAL TREATMENT

Surgical treatment of patients with CFM varies and no single surgical protocol exists for this condition. Functional impacts of CFM anomalies, such as upper airway obstruction, takes precedence and should be managed first if compromise exists. Although some investigators report success with neonatal mandible distraction osteogenesis (MDO), patients with CFM should be differentiated from those with RS because outcomes are generally less favorable in CFM than RS. In severe cases, tracheostomy may be required to secure the airway and was necessary in 35 of 755 patients treated in a multicenter study.[54]

In patients with airway obstruction, dysphagia, or both, a gastrostomy tube may be needed to provide the necessary nutrition requirements for a growing infant. These requirements are increased in patients with respiratory compromise owing to their increased work of breathing.

Correction of macrostomia and excision of branchial remnants is generally performed once the patient is felt safe for general anesthesia (6–

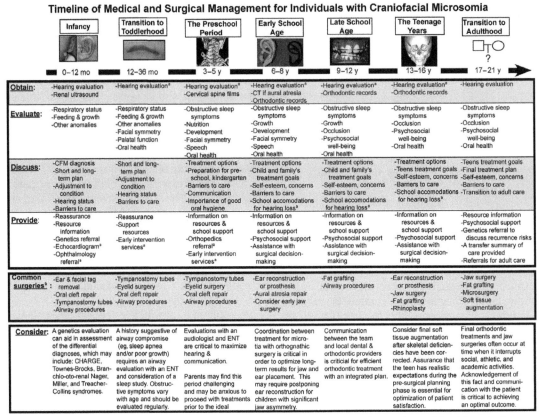

Timeline of Medical and Surgical Management for Individuals with Craniofacial Microsomia

	Infancy	Transition to Toddlerhood	The Preschool Period	Early School Age	Late School Age	The Teenage Years	Transition to Adulthood
	0–12 mo	12–36 mo	3–5 y	6–8 y	9–12 y	13–16 y	17–21 y
Obtain:	-Hearing evaluation -Renal ultrasound	-Hearing evaluation[a]	-Hearing evaluation[a] -Cervical spine films	-Hearing evaluation[a] -CT if aural atresia -Orthodontic records	-Hearing evaluation[a] -Orthodontic records	-Hearing evaluation[a] -Orthodontic records	-Hearing evaluation
Evaluate:	-Respiratory status -Feeding & growth -Other anomalies	-Respiratory status -Feeding & growth -Other anomalies -Facial symmetry -Palatal function -Oral health	-Obstructive sleep symptoms -Nutrition -Development -Facial symmetry -Speech -Oral health	-Obstructive sleep symptoms -Growth -Development -Facial symmetry -Speech -Oral health	-Obstructive sleep symptoms -Growth -Occlusion -Psychosocial well-being -Oral health	-Obstructive sleep symptoms -Occlusion -Psychosocial well-being -Oral health	-Obstructive sleep symptoms -Occlusion -Psychosocial well-being -Oral health
Discuss:	-CFM diagnosis -Short and long-term plan -Adjustment to condition -Hearing status -Barriers to care	-Short and long-term plan -Adjustment to condition -Hearing status -Barriers to care	-Treatment options -Preparation for pre-school, kindergarten -Barriers to care -Communication -Importance of good oral hygiene	-Treatment options -Child and family's treatment goals -Self-esteem, concerns -Barriers to care -School accomodations for hearing loss[a]	-Treatment options -Child and family's treatment goals -Self-esteem, concerns -Barriers to care -School accomodations for hearing loss[a]	-Treatment options -Teens treatment goals -Self-esteem, concerns -Barriers to care -School accomodations for hearing loss[b]	-Teens treatment goals -Final treatment plan -Self-esteem, concerns -Barriers to care -Transition to adult care
Provide:	-Reassurance -Resource information -Genetics referral -Echocardiogram[a] -Ophthalmology referral[a]	-Reassurance -Support resources -Early intervention services[a]	-Information on resources & school support -Orthopedics referral[a] -Early intervention services[a]	-Information on resources & school support -Psychosocial support -Assistance with surgical decision-making	-Information on resources & school support -Psychosocial support -Assistance with surgical decision-making	-Information on resources & school support -Psychosocial support -Assistance with surgical decision-making	-Resource information -Psychosocial support -Genetics referral to discuss recurrence risks -A transfer summary of care provided -Referrals for adult care
Common surgeries[b]:	-Ear & facial tag removal -Oral cleft repair -Tympanostomy tubes -Airway procedures	-Tympanostomy tubes -Eyelid surgery -Oral cleft repair -Airway procedures	-Tympanostomy tubes -Eyelid surgery -Oral cleft repair -Airway procedures	-Ear reconstruction or prosthesis -Aural atresia repair -Consider early jaw surgery	-Fat grafting -Airway procedures	-Ear reconstruction or prosthesis -Jaw surgery -Fat grafting -Rhinoplasty	-Jaw surgery -Fat grafting -Microsurgery -Soft tissue augmentation
Consider:	A genetics evaluation can aid in assessment of the differential diagnoses, which may include: CHARGE, Townes-Brocks, Branchio-oto-renal Nager, Miller, and Treacher-Collins syndromes.	A history suggestive of airway compromise (eg, sleep apnea and/or poor growth) requires an airway evaluation with an ENT and consideration of a sleep study. Obstructive symptoms vary with age and should be evaluated regularly.	Evaluations with an audiologist and ENT are critical to maximize hearing & communication. Parents may find this period challenging and may be anxious to proceed with treatments prior to the ideal	Coordination between treatment for micro-tia with orthognathic surgery is critical in order to optimize long-term results for jaw and ear placement. This may require postponing ear reconstruction for children with significant jaw asymmetry.	Communication between the team and local dental & orthodontic providers is criticial for efficient orthodontic treatment with an integrated plan.	Consider final soft tissue augmentation after skeletal deficiencies have been corrected. Assurance that the teen has realistic expectations during the pre-surgical planning phase is essential for optimization of patient satisfaction.	Final orthodontic treatments and jaw surgeries often occur at time when it interrupts social, athletic, and academic activities. Acknowledgement of this fact and communication with the patient is critical to achieving an optimal outcome.

Fig. 1. Timeline for care of patients with craniofacial microsomia (CFM). [a] When indicated. [b] Although these are common craniofacial surgeries in CFM, not all children will require every procedure.

12 months). Branchial remnants range from simple to complex and may be associated with the native underlying cartilage of the ear (**Fig. 3**). When excising these vestiges, it is important to remove any cartilaginous stalk at the remnant's base or this cartilage will continue to grow after excision of the superficial component. Macrostomia repair involves correction of the cleft within the mucosa

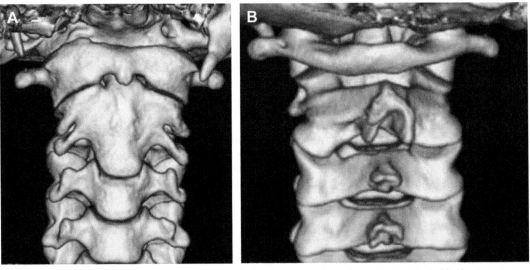

Fig. 2. Computed tomography scan displaying cervical spine anomalies of a patient with Goldenhar's variant of craniofacial microsomia (A) as compared with a normal control (B). Notice the fusion of C2 and C3 and dysmorphic dens.

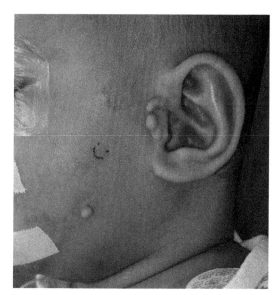

Fig. 3. Cheek and preauricular branchial remnants.

and cheek skin, but most important, recreation of the muscular sphincter of the mouth (**Fig. 4**).

Correction of orbital malposition generally involves elevating an orbit that is inferiorly displaced. Box osteotomies can be performed after the age of 6, once the orbital growth is complete.

Approaches to correction of the underdeveloped mandible in CFM are various and controversial. In general, Pruzansky I mandibles are managed with orthodontics and may not require surgical intervention. Divergence emerges with treatment of the Pruzansky IIa mandible. Some investigators report success of lengthening the shortened ramus with MDO with orthodontic management of the maxillary cant.[68–74] Others providers prefer awaiting skeletal maturity to perform bimaxillary orthognathic surgery.[75,76] For Pruzansky IIb mandibles, consideration of the TMJ dictates surgical approach. Classic descriptions involved simultaneous creation of a zygomatic arch and glenoid fossa with cranial bone grafts and conchal cartilage with ramus reconstruction using costochondral bone grafts.[77]

Concern over ankylosis has led many investigators to stage this reconstruction, whereas others have used MDO to lengthen the mandible ramus while using the skull base as a pseudo-TMJ without formal reconstruction. For Pruzansky III mandibles, a complete absence of mandible angle, ramus, and condyle require the addition of bony stock. Although some providers report success with MDO alone, other investigators recommend grafting before MDO.[78] A long history of success has been reported with costochondral bone grafting (**Fig. 5**), although the growth of this neoramus is variable.[79] More recently, vascularized free tissue transfer, typically a fibula free flap (**Fig. 6**), has been used to bring more robust bone and soft tissue to the deficient mandible,[80–83] although this too has been associated with ankylosis[84] and lacks growth potential.[85] No matter the technique, the goal of reconstruction is to create an adequate posterior ramus height and a functioning TMJ.

External ear reconstruction is another point of controversy. Although many surgical techniques exist for reconstructing grade 2 microtia, many surgeons prefer treating grades 2 and 3 microtic ears with a total ear reconstruction.[86] Options include prosthesis with an osseointegrated implant,[87,88] autologous rib graft reconstruction, and porous polyethylene.

Autologous reconstruction involves elevation of a skin flap, creation of a cartilage framework, lobule transposition, and creation of a postauricular sulcus. Generally, the surgery is performed between ages 6 and 10, once the ear has nearly reached adult size and the patient has enough costal cartilage to create an adult-sized framework. Various techniques have been described,[89–98] but most are grouped into either the Brent 3 stage approach[99,100] or the Nagata 2 stage approach.[101] The Brent technique requires less cartilage and can be performed any time after age 6. The contralateral synchondrosis of ribs 6 and 7 and cartilage of the eighth rib are used to create a construct similar to a template traced from the unaffected ear. Once carved, the

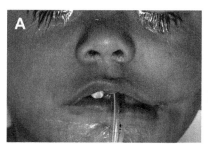
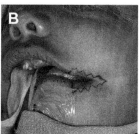
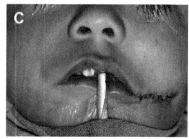

Fig. 4. Left-sided macrostomia preoperatively (*A*), intraoperatively with surgical markings including W-plasty (*B*), and after repair (*C*).

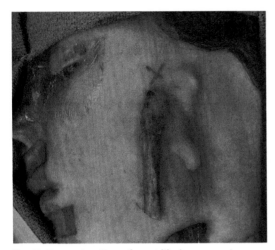

Fig. 5. Reconstruction of mandibular ramus in a patient with craniofacial microsomia and a Pruzansky III mandible using costochondral rib graft. The neoglenoid fossa is marked with an X based on preoperative planning and navigation.

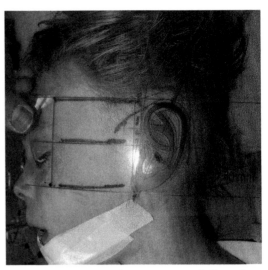

Fig. 7. Use of template for positioning of rib cartilage ear construct using the Nagata technique for microtia reconstruction.

construct is placed beneath the skin flap such that it lies symmetrically with the contralateral ear. A second stage involves lobule transposition and removal of any branchial vestiges, and the ear is then elevated in a third stage using a full-thickness skin graft to create a sulcus. The Nagata technique requires a larger cartilage construct and therefore is performed at an older age: generally age 10 or a chest circumference of at least 60 cm. With this technique, a standardized template is aligned with the superior and inferior orbital rims and cheek to locate the simultaneous skin flap elevation and lobule transposition (**Fig. 7**). The framework is carved from the cartilage of ribs 6, 7, 8 and 9 and is placed beneath the skin flap and around an attached area of skin, which will serve as the conchal bowl (**Fig. 8**). In a second stage, the framework is elevated from a postauricular incision and a temporoparietal fascia flap is wrapped around a wedge of banked cartilage

placed beneath and behind the framework to project the ear and create a sulcus. This fascia is then covered with either a split-thickness skin graft from the scalp or a full-thickness skin graft from the groin.

Although numerous materials have been used for alloplastic ear reconstruction,[102–106] porous polyethylene currently provides the best safety profile and is most widely used. Initial reports of extrusion, infection, and fracture slowed the acceptance of this technique, but more recent, long-term results seem to be favorable and have led to a greater acceptance.[107,108] Currently, 2 prefabricated constructs are available depending on patient characteristics, stability needs, and surgeon preference (**Fig. 9**). The construct is covered with a thin temporoparietal fascia flap and full-

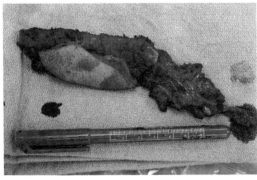

Fig. 6. Free fibula flap for reconstruction of the mandible ramus.

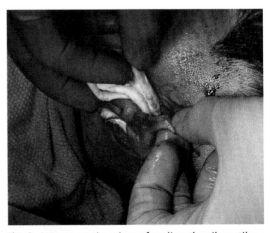

Fig. 8. Intraoperative view of curling the rib cartilage ear construct around the neoconchal bowl using the Nagata technique.

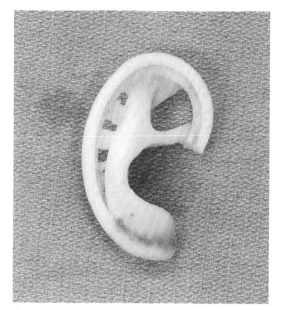

Fig. 9. MedPor ear implant after custom tailoring with strengthening buttresses.

thickness skin graft (**Fig. 10**). The advantages of alloplastic reconstruction include a lack of costal donor site, a single stage surgery, and the ability to perform the surgery at an earlier age, which may improve psychosocial acceptance.[109] Some centers are performing simultaneous external ear reconstruction with porous polyethylene and aural atresia reconstruction or placement of bone-anchored hearing aid,[110] and it seems to be an effective technique after aural atresia repair.[111]

Facial nerve palsy in CFM can be bilateral, but is more commonly unilateral and partial. When considering facial reanimation surgery, one must

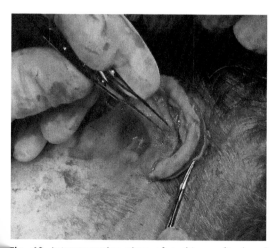

Fig. 10. Intraoperative view of a skin graft placed over the temporoparietal fascia flap in MedPor ear reconstruction.

first consider the patient's ability to protect the cornea from dryness, which can lead to ulceration and blindness. Daily drops and nightly ointment may suffice, but some patients prefer a surgical solution. Although tarsorrhaphies can be effective,[112] they are unsightly. The combination of a gold[113] or platinum[114] weight to the upper eyelid and a lower eyelid sling has been shown to be effective[115] (**Fig. 11**). Although the brow will eventually descend with age and force of gravity, treatment generally is not necessary in the pediatric patient with CFM, but is more likely reserved for adults with frontal branch palsy. Similarly, although static procedures with alloplastic[116] or autogenous slings[117] are common in adults, the pediatric patient with CFM will generally benefit more from dynamic reanimation procedures.

The most common dynamic procedure performed in patients with CFM and unilateral facial palsy is the 2-stage facial reanimation procedure. In this procedure, a cross-face nerve graft using the sural nerve as a donor is placed from a redundant buccal branch of the normative side and strung across the face to the affected side, where its distal end is placed in the upper lip (**Fig. 12**). There, it is connected to a sensory branch of the infraorbital nerve to promote growth. After awaiting ingrowth (3–6 months), a biopsy is performed to confirm axonal ingrowth and stage 2 proceeds with a microvascular muscle transfer. Although many donor muscles have been described, the gracilis is favored owing to its predictable anatomy, length of neurovascular pedicle, and ability to use a 2-team approach.[118] The advantage of the 2-stage reanimation procedure is the ability to create a spontaneous smile. The disadvantages are the need for 2 stages separated by many months, placement of scar on the unaffected side, and weaker smile generated. For this reason, some surgeons prefer alternate approaches. Locoregional muscle flaps such as the masseter[119] and temporalis[120–122] share the benefit of single-side surgery with no delay for dynamic function. However, although improved static tone is seen, the lack of dynamic strength and temporal hollowing[123] are among criticisms for this technique. Postoperative measurements of facial movement[124] have indicated good overall results and newer technologies are being developed to document this return of function.[125]

Although a great deal of emphasis has been placed on bony reconstruction in CFM, the soft tissue deficiency is an important component of CFM and should be addressed in conjunction to any bony work. Orofacial clefts at the philtrum are uncommon and can be treated following the protocol of typical cleft care. More commonly, lateral facial

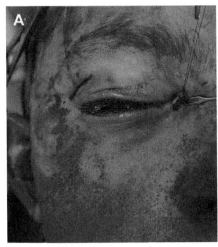
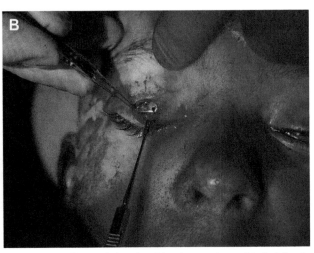

Fig. 11. (*A*) Palmaris longus lower eyelid sling for correction of lower lid malposition in a patient with facial palsy. (*B*) Gold weight placement to upper eyelid for treatment of lagophthalmos in a patient with facial palsy.

clefts at the commissure (Tessier VII clefts of mascrostomia) are present in CFM and require treatment with commissuroplasty. Numerous techniques exist, but the goals include (1) normalizing the commissure position, (2) repairing the mucosa with a local flap, (3) reconstructing the orbicularis oris muscle in a vest over pants fashion, and (4) minimizing facial scarring.[126]

Soft tissue deficiency can be camouflaged with alloplastic implants such as porous polyethylene,[127,128] some of which can be designed

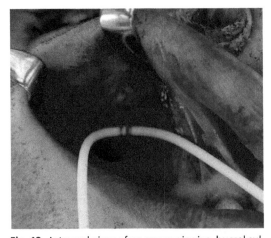

Fig. 12. Intraoral view of an upper gingiva–buccal sulcus approach during the first stage of a facial reanimation procedure (cross-face nerve graft). A neurorrhaphy is performed to a buccal branch and the distal end of the sural nerve graft is tunneled to the contralateral lip. Here, a vessel loop identifies a branch of the infraorbital nerve in the lip to which an additional neurorrhaphy is performed to improve axonal ingrowth.

individually for patient-specific needs.[129] However, many patients will require soft tissue augmentation with local flaps, distant flaps, dermal fat grafts, or structural fat grafting. Local flaps are limited in availability, but dermal fat grafts and free flaps can be designed all over the body where blood supply is adequate and donor scarring will be less conspicuous. Numerous free flaps have been described for treatment of CFM[130–134] and are generally reserved for more severe cases.[80,135] Owing to the robust blood supply brought with the free flap, revisions tend to involve debulking procedures (**Fig. 13**). Dermal fat grafts are not limited by blood supply, but tend to resorb and revisions tend to require additional augmentation.[136] In many ways, structural fat grafting has supplanted these techniques for soft tissue augmentation in CFM.[137,138] The benefit of microfat injections is the limited scarring, minimal donor site morbidity, ability to attain precise augmentation, and the preservation of the retaining ligaments of the face. It can be performed as a brief outpatient procedure or combined with other procedures such as microtia reconstruction or dental work.

Many patients with CFM will benefit from orthognathic surgery to level their occlusal cant and improve their skeletal asymmetry. Ideally, this definitive orthognathic surgery is postponed until skeletal maturity to decrease the need for repeat surgery. Often, orthognathic surgery in this patient population involves both jaws, the movement of which is more complex than straightforward advancements or setbacks (**Fig. 14**). For this reason, precise preoperative planning is crucial. Conventional planning with cephalometric tracings, stone model surgery, and an articulator

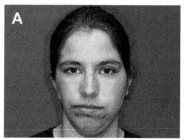 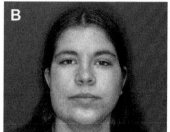 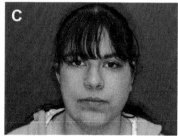

Fig. 13. Soft tissue reconstruction in craniofacial microsomia with free flaps often require debulking revisions. Preoperative photo of patient with right lower face deficiency (*A*). Postoperative photo after soft tissue augmentation with free groin flap (*B*). Postoperative photo after debulking of free flap displaying improved contour and symmetry (*C*).

remains the gold standard. However, many surgeons prefer virtual surgical planning for these complex cases.[139–143] Its benefits include ease of manipulating the segments, ability to trial multiple surgical techniques, detection of areas of interference, and postoperative measurements at various points that can be correlated intraoperatively (**Table 3**).

RESEARCH OPPORTUNITIES

We have little evidence for many of the current recommendations for care in individuals with CFM. A lack of understanding about etiology, the absence of consensus on diagnostic criteria, and a paucity of large population studies have hampered our ability to make significant advances in the requisite research required to provide robust, evidence-based treatment guidelines.

In 2009, the Facial Asymmetry Collaborative for Interdisciplinary Assessment and Learning (FACIAL) was formed to develop a multicenter research infrastructure to facilitate research in CFM. The FACIAL network established research eligibility criteria that required participants to have at least one of the features described in **Box 1** and, in addition, an absence of other characteristics associated with established syndromes with overlapping features of CFM. The network continues to expand, and goals include further investigation of the genetic contributions to CFM through Dr Luquetti's partnership with the National Institutes of Health Gabriella Miller Kids First Program and interdisciplinary collaboration to investigate patient preferences and clinical outcomes.

The International Consortium for Health Outcome Metrics working group for CFM (https://www.ichom.org/medical-conditions/craniofacial-microsomia/) developed a set of outcome metrics related to the following domains: functioning, appearance, psychosocial, and treatment burden. Recent publications provide a call to

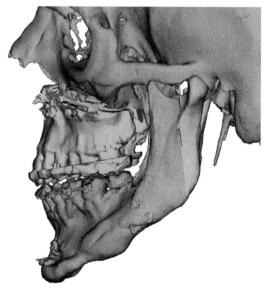

Fig. 14. Virtual surgical plan for 2-jaw surgery in patient with skeletal asymmetry and occlusal cant secondary to craniofacial microsomia.

Box 1
Minimal inclusion criteria for clinical research proposed by the Facial Asymmetry Collaborative for Interdisciplinary Assessment and Learning research network

- Microtia/anotia
- Facial asymmetry + preauricular tag(s)
- Facial asymmetry + facial tag(s)
- Facial asymmetry + epibulbar dermoid
- Facial asymmetry + macrostomia
- Preauricular tag + epibulbar dermoid
- Preauricular tag + macrostomia
- Facial tag + epibulbar dermoid
- Macrostomia + epibulbar dermoid

Table 3
Predicted surgical movement at facial landmarks based on virtual surgical planning

Point	Name	Anterior/Posterior	Left/Right	Up/Down
ANS	Anterior nasal spine	5.40 mm anterior	0.02 mm right	1.86 mm up
A	A point	5.11 mm anterior	1.66 mm right	1.98 mm up
ISU1	Midline of upper incisor	5.00 mm anterior	3.00 mm right	2.00 mm up
U3L	Upper left canine	7.13 mm anterior	1.30 mm right	0.64 mm up
U6L	Upper left anterior molar (mesiobuccal cusp)	7.79 mm anterior	0.66 mm left	0.28 mm up
U3R	Upper right canine	2.24 mm anterior	1.15 mm right	3.93 mm up
U6R	Upper right anterior molar (mesiobuccal cusp)	1.52 mm anterior	0.69 mm left	4.49 mm up
ISL1	Midline of lower incisor	1.95 mm anterior	5.55 mm left	3.38 mm up
L6L	Lower left anterior molar (mesiobuccal cusp)	1.02 mm anterior	5.18 mm left	2.14 mm up
L6R	Lower right anterior molar (mesiobuccal cusp)	2.86 mm anterior	4.77 mm left	3.94 mm up
B	B point	2.54 mm anterior	4.10 mm left	3.19 mm up
Pog	Pogonion	2.86 mm anterior	3.64 mm left	3.28 mm up

Intraoperative measurements at these points can be made to confirm appropriate surgical movement.

action for further investigation of the psychosocial needs of individuals with CFM,[53,144–146] and identification of optimal screening tools and intervention strategies, when indicated.

CONTROVERSIES

The treatment of children with CFM should be performed in collaboration with a craniofacial team and based on the patient's needs and personal preferences. We have opportunities to significantly improve the existing research base by addressing many current treatment controversies. For patients with Pruzansky III mandibles, is it more effective to perform distraction osteogenesis, costochondral grafting, and/or free fibula flaps? For individuals who lack the glenoid fossa, is it best to simultaneously reconstruct the glenoid and condyle, or perform a staged approach? For individuals with a Pruzansky II mandible, are long-term outcomes more favorable when completing mandibular distraction osteogenesis during mixed dentition with orthodontic manipulation of the maxilla, or with a 2-jaw surgery at skeletal maturity? Are patients with microtia more satisfied with the long-term outcomes of external ear reconstruction with autologous rib graft constructs or porous polyethylene? Additionally, the simultaneous creation of an external auditory canal for patients with microtia and aural atresia remains controversial. In the end, an approach that optimizes final facial symmetry while minimizing

surgical interventions and remains sensitive to patients' social and self-confidence needs is one that best serves the patient with CFM.

REFERENCES

1. Bennun RD, Mulliken JB, Kaban LB, et al. Microtia: a microform of hemifacial microsomia. Plast Reconstr Surg 1985;76:859–65.
2. Converse JM, Coccaro PJ, Becker M, et al. On hemifacial microsomia. The first and second branchial arch syndrome. Plast Reconstr Surg 1973;51:268–79.
3. Rollnick BR, Kaye CI. Hemifacial microsomia and variants: pedigree data. Am J Med Genet 1983;15:233–53.
4. Stark RB, Saunders DE. The first branchial syndrome. The oral-mandibular-auricular syndrome. Plast Reconstr Surg Transplant Bull 1962;29:229–39.
5. Cohen MM Jr, Rollnick BR, Kaye CI. Oculoauriculovertebral spectrum: an updated critique. Cleft Palate J 1989;26:276–86.
6. Poswillo D. The aetiology and pathogenesis of craniofacial deformity. Development 1988;103 Suppl:207–12.
7. Grabb WC. The first and second branchial arch syndrome. Plast Reconstr Surg 1965;36:485–508.
8. Ohtani J, Hoffman WY, Vargervik K, et al. Team management and treatment outcomes for patients with hemifacial microsomia. Am J Orthod Dentofacial Orthop 2012;141:S74–81.

9. Farina R, Valladares S, Torrealba R, et al. Orthognathic surgery in craniofacial microsomia: treatment algorithm. Plast Reconstr Surg Glob Open 2015;3:e294.

10. Johnston MC, Bronsky PT. Prenatal craniofacial development: new insights on normal and abnormal mechanisms. Crit Rev Oral Biol Med 1995;6:368–422.

11. Johnston MC, Bronsky PT. Animal models for human craniofacial malformations. J Craniofac Genet Dev Biol 1991;11:277–91.

12. Poswillo D. The pathogenesis of the first and second branchial arch syndrome. Oral Surg Oral Med Oral Pathol 1973;35:302–28.

13. Werler MM, Sheehan JE, Hayes C, et al. Demographic and reproductive factors associated with hemifacial microsomia. Cleft Palate Craniofac J 2004;41. https://doi.org/10.1597/03-110.1.

14. Werler MM, Sheehan JE, Hayes C, et al. Vasoactive exposures, vascular events, and hemifacial microsomia. Birth Defects Res A Clin Mol Teratol 2004;70:389–95.

15. Padwa BL, Bruneteau RJ, Mulliken JB. Association between "plagiocephaly" and hemifacial microsomia. Am J Med Genet 1993;47:1202–7.

16. Fryns JP, Lemaire J, Timmermans J, et al. The association of hemifacial microsomia, homolateral micro/anophthalmos, hemihypotrophy, dental anomalies, submucous cleft palate, CNS malformations and hypopigmented skin lesions following Blaschko's lines in two unrelated female patients. Further evidence for a lethal mutation surviving in mosaic form in "hypomelanosis of Ito. Genet Couns 1993; 4:63–7.

17. Beals RK, Robbins JR, Rolfe B. Anomalies associated with vertebral malformations. Spine (Phila Pa 1976) 1993;18:1329–32.

18. Duncan PA, Shapiro LR. Interrelationships of the hemifacial microsomia-VATER, VATER, and sirenomelia phenotypes. Am J Med Genet 1993;47:75–84.

19. Kaye CI, Martin AO, Rollnick BR, et al. Oculoauriculovertebral anomaly: segregation analysis. Am J Med Genet 1992;43:913–7.

20. Taysi K, Marsh JL, Wise DM. Familial hemifacial microsomia. Cleft Palate J 1983;20:47–53.

21. Juriloff DM, Harris MJ, Froster-Iskenius U. Hemifacial deficiency induced by a shift in dominance of the mouse mutation far: a possible genetic model for hemifacial microsomia. J Craniofac Genet Dev Biol 1987;7:27–44.

22. Poonawalla HH, Kaye CI, Rosenthal IM, et al. Hemifacial microsomia in a patient with Klinefelter syndrome. Cleft Palate J 1980;17:194–6.

23. Kaye CI, Rollnick BR, Pruzansky S. Malformations of the auricle: isolated and in syndromes. IV. Cumulative pedigree data. Birth Defects Orig Artic Ser 1979;15:163–9.

24. Smahel Z. Craniofacial changes in hemifacial microsomia. J Craniofac Genet Dev Biol 1986;6: 151–70.

25. Zielinski D, Markus B, Sheikh M, et al. OTX2 duplication is implicated in hemifacial microsomia. PLoS One 2014;9:e96788.

26. Guida V, Sinibaldi L, Pagnoni M, et al. A de novo proximal 3q29 chromosome microduplication in a patient with oculo auriculo vertebral spectrum. Am J Med Genet A 2015;167A:797–801.

27. Beleza-Meireles A, Clayton-Smith J, Saraiva JM, et al. Oculo-auriculo-vertebral spectrum: a review of the literature and genetic update. J Med Genet 2014;51:635–45.

28. Xu J, Fan YS, Siu VM. A child with features of Goldenhar syndrome and a novel 1.12 Mb deletion in 22q11.2 by cytogenetics and oligonucleotide array CGH: is this a candidate region for the syndrome? Am J Med Genet A 2008;146A:1886–9.

29. Digilio MC, McDonald-McGinn DM, Heike C, et al. Three patients with oculo-auriculo-vertebral spectrum and microdeletion 22q11.2. Am J Med Genet A 2009;149A:2860–4.

30. Tan TY, Collins A, James PA, et al. Phenotypic variability of distal 22q11.2 copy number abnormalities. Am J Med Genet A 2011;155A:1623–33.

31. Cousley RR. A comparison of two classification systems for hemifacial microsomia. Br J Oral Maxillofac Surg 1993;31:78–82.

32. Purnell CA, Janes LE, Klosowiak JL, et al. Mandibular catch-up growth in Pierre Robin sequence: a systematic review. Cleft Palate Craniofac J 2018. https://doi.org/10.1177/1055665618774025.

33. Evans AK, Rahbar R, Rogers GF, et al. Robin sequence: a retrospective review of 115 patients. Int J Pediatr Otorhinolaryngol 2006;70:973–80.

34. Pruzansky S. Not all dwarfed mandibles are alike. Birth Defects 1969;1:120–9.

35. Kaban LB, Moses MH, Mulliken JB. Surgical correction of hemifacial microsomia in the growing child. Plast Reconstr Surg 1988;82:9–19.

36. Kaban LB, Mulliken JB, Murray JE. Three-dimensional approach to analysis and treatment of hemifacial microsomia. Cleft Palate J 1981;18:90–9.

37. Steinbacher DM, Gougoutas A, Bartlett SP. An analysis of mandibular volume in hemifacial microsomia. Plast Reconstr Surg 2011;127:2407–12.

38. Bartlett SP, Taylor JA, Goldstein JA, et al. Reply: mandibular deformity in hemifacial microsomia: a reassessment of the Pruzansky and Kaban classification. Plast Reconstr Surg 2014;134:658e–9e.

39. Wink JD, Goldstein JA, Paliga JT, et al. The mandibular deformity in hemifacial microsomia: a reassessment of the Pruzansky and Kaban classification. Plast Reconstr Surg 2014;133:174e–81e.

40. Swanson JW, Mitchell BT, Wink JA, et al. Surgical classification of the mandibular deformity in

craniofacial microsomia using 3-dimensional computed tomography. Plast Reconstr Surg Glob Open 2016;4:e598.

41. Converse JM, Wood-Smith D, McCarthy JG, et al. Bilateral facial microsomia. Diagnosis, classification, treatment. Plast Reconstr Surg 1974;54:413–23.

42. Figueroa AA, Pruzansky S. The external ear, mandible and other components of hemifacial microsomia. J Maxillofac Surg 1982;10:200–11.

43. Longacre JJ. The surgical management of the first and second branchial arch syndrome. Br J Plast Surg 1965;18:243–53.

44. Lauritzen C, Munro IR, Ross RB. Classification and treatment of hemifacial microsomia. Scand J Plast Reconstr Surg 1985;19:33–9.

45. David DJ, Mahatumarat C, Cooter RD. Hemifacial microsomia: a multisystem classification. Plast Reconstr Surg 1987;80:525–35.

46. Vento AR, LaBrie RA, Mulliken JB. The O.M.E.N.S. classification of hemifacial microsomia. Cleft Palate Craniofac J 1991;28:68–76 [discussion: 77].

47. Horgan JE, Padwa BL, LaBrie RA, et al. OMENS-Plus: analysis of craniofacial and extracraniofacial anomalies in hemifacial microsomia. Cleft Palate Craniofac J 1995;32:405–12.

48. Gougoutas AJ, Singh DJ, Low DW, et al. Hemifacial microsomia: clinical features and pictographic representations of the OMENS classification system. Plast Reconstr Surg 2007;120:112e–20e.

49. Birgfeld CB, Luquetti DV, Gougoutas AJ, et al. A phenotypic assessment tool for craniofacial microsomia. Plast Reconstr Surg 2011;127:313–20.

50. Tuin AJ, Tahiri Y, Paine KM, et al. Clarifying the relationships among the different features of the OMENS+ classification in craniofacial microsomia. Plast Reconstr Surg 2015;135:149e–56e.

51. Speltz ML, Kapp-Simon KA, Johns AL, et al. Neurodevelopment of Infants with and without craniofacial microsomia. J Pediatr 2018;198:226–33.e3.

52. Stock NM, Feragen KB. Comparing psychological adjustment across cleft and other craniofacial conditions: implications for outcome measurement and intervention. Cleft Palate Craniofac J 2018. https://doi.org/10.1177/1055665618770183.

53. Johns AL, Luquetti DV, Brajcich MR, et al. In their own words: caregiver and patient perspectives on stressors, resources, and recommendations in craniofacial microsomia care. J Craniofac Surg 2018;29:2198–205.

54. Caron CJJM, Pluijmers BI, Maas BDPJ, et al. Obstructive sleep apnoea in craniofacial microsomia: analysis of 755 patients. Int J Oral Maxillofac Surg 2017;46:1330–7.

55. van de Lande LS, Caron CJJM, Pluijmers BI, et al. Evaluation of swallow function in patients with craniofacial microsomia: a retrospective study. Dysphagia 2018;33:234–42.

56. Matsuo K, Palmer JB. Anatomy and physiology of feeding and swallowing: normal and abnormal. Phys Med Rehabil Clin N Am 2008;19:691–707, vii.

57. Cohen MS, Samango-Sprouse CA, Stern HJ, et al. Neurodevelopmental profile of infants and toddlers with oculo-auriculo-vertebral spectrum and the correlation of prognosis with physical findings. Am J Med Genet 1995;60:535–40.

58. Frisdal A, Trainor PA. Development and evolution of the pharyngeal apparatus. Wiley Interdiscip Rev Dev Biol 2014;3:403–18.

59. Huisinga-Fischer CE, Zonneveld FW, Vaandrager JM, et al. Relationship in hypoplasia between the masticatory muscles and the craniofacial skeleton in hemifacial microsomia, as determined by 3-D CT imaging. J Craniofac Surg 2001;12:31–40.

60. Miller CK. Feeding issues and interventions in infants and children with clefts and craniofacial syndromes. Semin Speech Lang 2011;32:115–26.

61. Rajendran T, Ramalinggam G, Kamaru Ambu V. Rare presentation of bilobed posterior tongue in Goldenhar syndrome. BMJ Case Rep 2017. https://doi.org/10.1136/bcr-2017-219726.

62. Chen EH, Reid RR, Chike-Obi C, et al. Tongue dysmorphology in craniofacial microsomia. Plast Reconstr Surg 2009;124:583–9.

63. Birgfeld CB, Heike CL, Saltzman BS, et al. Reliable classification of facial phenotypic variation in craniofacial microsomia: a comparison of physical exam and photographs. Head Face Med 2016; 12:14.

64. Caron CJJM, Pluijmers BI, Wolvius EB, et al. Craniofacial and extracraniofacial anomalies in craniofacial microsomia: a multicenter study of 755 patients. J Craniomaxillofac Surg 2017;45: 1302–10.

65. Goldenhar M. Associations malformatives de loeil et de loreille en particulier le syndrome dermoide epibulbare-appendices auriculaires-fistula auris congenita et ses relations avec la dysostose mandibulofacial. J Genet Hum 1952;1:343–82.

66. Konas E, Canter HI, Mavili ME. Goldenhar complex with atypical associated anomalies: is the spectrum still widening? J Craniofac Surg 2006;17: 669–72.

67. Tuin J, Tahiri Y, Paliga JT, et al. Distinguishing Goldenhar syndrome from craniofacial microsomia. J Craniofac Surg 2015;26:1887–92.

68. Kaban LB, Padwa BL, Mulliken JB. Surgical correction of mandibular hypoplasia in hemifacial microsomia: the case for treatment in early childhood. J Oral Maxillofac Surg 1998;56:628–38.

69. Weichman KE, Jacobs J, Patel P, et al. Early distraction for mild to moderate unilateral craniofacial microsomia: long-term follow-up, outcomes, and recommendations. Plast Reconstr Surg 2017; 139:941e–53e.

70. Kearns GJ, Padwa BL, Mulliken JB, et al. Progression of facial asymmetry in hemifacial microsomia. Plast Reconstr Surg 2000;105:492–8.

71. Meazzini MC, Mazzoleni F, Gabriele C, et al. Mandibular distraction osteogenesis in hemifacial microsomia: long-term follow-up. J Craniomaxillofac Surg 2005;33:370–6.

72. James D, Ma L. Mandibular reconstruction in children with obstructive sleep apnea due to micrognathia. Plast Reconstr Surg 1997;100:1131–7 [discussion: 1138].

73. Singh DJ, Glick PH, Bartlett SP. Mandibular deformities: single-vector distraction techniques for a multivector problem. J Craniofac Surg 2009;20: 1468–72.

74. McCarthy JG, Katzen JT, Hopper R, et al. The first decade of mandibular distraction: lessons we have learned. Plast Reconstr Surg 2002;110:1704–13.

75. Ko EW, Chen PK, Lo LJ. Comparison of the adult three-dimensional craniofacial features of patients with unilateral craniofacial microsomia with and without early mandible distraction. Int J Oral Maxillofac Surg 2017;46:811–8.

76. Nagy K, Kuijpers-Jagtman AM, Mommaerts MY. No evidence for long-term effectiveness of early osteodistraction in hemifacial microsomia. Plast Reconstr Surg 2009;124:2061–71.

77. Munro IR, Lauritzen CG. Classification and treatment of hemifacial microsomia. In: Carroni EP, editor. Craniofacial Surgery. Boston: Little, Brown & Co; 1985. p. 391–400.

78. Wan DC, Taub PJ, Allam KA, et al. Distraction osteogenesis of costocartilaginous rib grafts and treatment algorithm for severely hypoplastic mandibles. Plast Reconstr Surg 2011;127: 2005–13.

79. Tahiri Y, Chang CS, Tuin J, et al. Costochondral grafting in craniofacial microsomia. Plast Reconstr Surg 2015;135:530–41.

80. Siebert JW, Anson G, Longaker MT. Microsurgical correction of facial asymmetry in 60 consecutive cases. Plast Reconstr Surg 1996;97:354–63.

81. Warren SM, Borud LJ, Brecht LE, et al. Microvascular reconstruction of the pediatric mandible. Plast Reconstr Surg 2007;119:649–61.

82. Santamaria E, Morales C, Taylor JA, et al. Mandibular microsurgical reconstruction in patients with hemifacial microsomia. Plast Reconstr Surg 2008; 122:1839–49.

83. Cleveland EC, Zampell J, Avraham T, et al. Reconstruction of Congenital mandibular hypoplasia with microvascular free fibula flaps in the pediatric population: a paradigm shift. J Craniofac Surg 2017; 28:79–83.

84. Resnick CM, Genuth J, Calabrese CE, et al. Temporomandibular joint ankylosis after ramus construction with free fibula flaps in children with hemifacial microsomia. J Oral Maxillofac Surg 2018. https://doi.org/10.1016/j.joms.2018.05.004.

85. Zhang WB, Liang T, Peng X. Mandibular growth after paediatric mandibular reconstruction with the vascularized free fibula flap: a systematic review. Int J Oral Maxillofac Surg 2016;45:440–7. https://doi.org/10.1016/j.ijom.2015.12.014.

86. Bauer BS. Reconstruction of the microtic ear. J Pediatr Surg 1984;19:440–5.

87. Ryan MA, Khoury T, Kaylie DM, et al. Osseointegrated implants for auricular prostheses: an alternative to autologous repair. Laryngoscope 2018. https://doi.org/10.1002/lary.27128.

88. Tjellstrom A. Osseointegrated implants for replacement of absent or defective ears. Clin Plast Surg 1990;17:355–66.

89. Tanzer RC. Total reconstruction of the external ear. Plast Reconstr Surg Transplant Bull 1959; 23:1–15.

90. Walton RL, Beahm EK. Auricular reconstruction for microtia: part II. Surgical techniques. Plast Reconstr Surg 2002;110:234–49 [quiz: 250–1], 387.

91. Beahm EK, Walton RL. Auricular reconstruction for microtia: part I. Anatomy, embryology, and clinical evaluation. Plast Reconstr Surg 2002;109: 2473–82 [quiz: 2482].

92. Nagata S. Modification of the stages in total reconstruction of the auricle: part IV. Ear elevation for the constructed auricle. Plast Reconstr Surg 1994;93: 254–66 [discussion: 267–8].

93. Nagata S. Modification of the stages in total reconstruction of the auricle: part III. Grafting the three-dimensional costal cartilage framework for small concha-type microtia. Plast Reconstr Surg 1994; 93:243–53 [discussion: 267–8].

94. Nagata S. Modification of the stages in total reconstruction of the auricle: part II. Grafting the three-dimensional costal cartilage framework for concha-type microtia. Plast Reconstr Surg 1994; 93:231–42 [discussion: 267–8].

95. Nagata S. Modification of the stages in total reconstruction of the auricle: part I. Grafting the three-dimensional costal cartilage framework for lobule-type microtia. Plast Reconstr Surg 1994;93: 221–30 [discussion: 267–8].

96. Cho BC, Kim JY, Byun JS. Two-stage reconstruction of the auricle in congenital microtia using autogenous costal cartilage. J Plast Reconstr Aesthet Surg 2007;60:998–1006.

97. Pan B, Jiang H, Guo D, et al. Microtia: ear reconstruction using tissue expander and autogenous costal cartilage. J Plast Reconstr Aesthet Surg 2008;61(Suppl 1):S98–103.

98. Firmin F. Auricular reconstruction in cases of microtia. Principles, methods and classification. Ann Chir Plast Esthet 2001;46:447–66 [in French].

99. Brent B. Microtia repair with rib cartilage grafts: a review of personal experience with 1000 cases. Clin Plast Surg 2002;29:257–71, vii.

100. Brent B. Auricular repair with autogenous rib cartilage grafts: two decades of experience with 600 cases. Plast Reconstr Surg 1992;90:355–74 [discussion: 375–6].

101. Nagata S. A new method of total reconstruction of the auricle for microtia. Plast Reconstr Surg 1993; 92:187–201.

102. Lynch JB, Pousti A, Doyle JE, et al. Our experiences with silastic ear implants. Plast Reconstr Surg 1972;49:283–5.

103. Reinisch JF, Lewin S. Ear reconstruction using a porous polyethylene framework and temporoparietal fascia flap. Facial Plast Surg 2009;25:181–9.

104. Wellisz T. Clinical experience with the Medpor porous polyethylene implant. Aesthetic Plast Surg 1993;17:339–44.

105. Baluch N, Nagata S, Park C, et al. Auricular reconstruction for microtia: a review of available methods. Plast Surg (Oakv) 2014;22:39–43.

106. Yang SL, Zheng JH, Ding Z, et al. Combined fascial flap and expanded skin flap for enveloping Medpor framework in microtia reconstruction. Aesthetic Plast Surg 2009;33:518–22.

107. Harii K, Asato H, Yoshimura K, et al. One-stage transfer of the latissimus dorsi muscle for reanimation of a paralyzed face: a new alternative. Plast Reconstr Surg 1998;102:941–51.

108. Reinisch J, Tahiri Y. Polyethylene ear reconstruction: a state-of-the-art surgical journey. Plast Reconstr Surg 2018;141:461–70.

109. Horlock N, Vogelin E, Bradbury ET, et al. Psychosocial outcome of patients after ear reconstruction: a retrospective study of 62 patients. Ann Plast Surg 2005;54:517–24.

110. Romo T 3rd, Morris LG, Reitzen SD, et al. Reconstruction of congenital microtia-atresia: outcomes with the Medpor/bone-anchored hearing aid-approach. Ann Plast Surg 2009;62:384–9.

111. Roberson JB Jr, Reinisch J, Colen TY, et al. Atresia repair before microtia reconstruction: comparison of early with standard surgical timing. Otol Neurotol 2009;30:771–6.

112. Maas CS, Benecke JE, Holds JB, et al. Primary surgical management for rehabilitation of the paralyzed eye. Otolaryngol Head Neck Surg 1994; 110:288–95.

113. Rofagha S, Seiff SR. Long-term results for the use of gold eyelid load weights in the management of facial paralysis. Plast Reconstr Surg 2010;125: 142–9.

114. Silver AL, Lindsay RW, Cheney ML, et al. Thin-profile platinum eyelid weighting: a superior option in the paralyzed eye. Plast Reconstr Surg 2009;123: 1697–703.

115. Terzis JK, Kyere SA. Minitendon graft transfer for suspension of the paralyzed lower eyelid: our experience. Plast Reconstr Surg 2008;121: 1206–16.

116. Skourtis ME, Weber SM, Kriet JD, et al. Immediate Gore-Tex sling suspension for management of facial paralysis in head and neck extirpative surgery. Otolaryngol Head Neck Surg 2007;137: 228–32.

117. Rose EH. Autogenous fascia lata grafts: clinical applications in reanimation of the totally or partially paralyzed face. Plast Reconstr Surg 2005;116: 20–32 [discussion: 33–5].

118. Sharma PR, Zuker RM, Borschel GH. Gracilis free muscle transfer in the treatment of pediatric facial paralysis. Facial Plast Surg 2016;32:199–208.

119. Baker DC, Conley J. Regional muscle transposition for rehabilitation of the paralyzed face. Clin Plast Surg 1979;6:317–31.

120. Labbe D, Huault M. Lengthening temporalis myoplasty and lip reanimation. Plast Reconstr Surg 2000;105:1289–97 [discussion: 1298].

121. Sidle DM, Fishman AJ. Modification of the orthodromic temporalis tendon transfer technique for reanimation of the paralyzed face. Otolaryngol Head Neck Surg 2011;145:18–23.

122. May M, Drucker C. Temporalis muscle for facial reanimation. A 13-year experience with 224 procedures. Arch Otolaryngol Head Neck Surg 1993; 119:378–82 [discussion: 383–4].

123. Bos R, Reddy SG, Mommaerts MY. Lengthening temporalis myoplasty versus free muscle transfer with the gracilis flap for long-standing facial paralysis: a systematic review of outcomes. J Craniomaxillofac Surg 2016;44:940–51.

124. Manktelow RT, Zuker RM, Tomat LR. Facial paralysis measurement with a handheld ruler. Plast Reconstr Surg 2008;121:435–42.

125. Hammal Z, Cohn JF, Wallace ER, et al. Facial expressiveness in infants with and without craniofacial microsomia: preliminary findings. Cleft Palate Craniofac J 2018;55:711–20.

126. Tahiri Y, Birgfeld C, Bartlett S. Plastic surgery. In: Neligan P, editor. Ch. Craniofacial microsomia, vol. 3, 4th edition. Elsevier; 2018. p. 774–800.

127. Seo JS, Roh YC, Song JM, et al. Sequential treatment for a patient with hemifacial microsomia: 10 year-long term follow up. Maxillofac Plast Reconstr Surg 2015;37:3.

128. Andrade NN, Raikwar K. Medpor in maxillofacial deformities: report of three cases. J Maxillofac Oral Surg 2009;8:192–5.

129. Staal F, Pluijmers B, Wolvius E, et al. Patient-specific implant for residual facial asymmetry following orthognathic surgery in unilateral craniofacial microsomia. Craniomaxillofac Trauma Reconstr 2016;9:264–7.

130. Siebert JW, Longaker MT, Angrigiani C. The infra-mammary extended circumflex scapular flap: an aesthetic improvement of the parascapular flap. Plast Reconstr Surg 1997;99:70–7.

131. Anderl H. Free vascularized groin fat flap in hypoplasia and hemiatrophy of the face (a three years observation). J Maxillofac Surg 1979;7:327–32.

132. Cooper TM, Lewis N, Baldwin MA. Free groin flap revisited. Plast Reconstr Surg 1999;103:918–24.

133. Jurkiewicz MJ, Nahai F. The omentum: its use as a free vascularized graft for reconstruction of the head and neck. Ann Surg 1982;195:756–65.

134. Tuncali D, Baser NT, Terzioglu A, et al. Romberg's disease associated with Horner's syndrome: contour restoration by a free anterolateral thigh perforator flap and ancillary procedures. Plast Reconstr Surg 2007;120:67e–72e.

135. Longaker MT, Siebert JW. Microsurgical correction of facial contour in congenital craniofacial malformations: the marriage of hard and soft tissue. Plast Reconstr Surg 1996;98:942–50.

136. Mordick TG 2nd, Larossa D, Whitaker L. Soft-tissue reconstruction of the face: a comparison of dermal-fat grafting and vascularized tissue transfer. Ann Plast Surg 1992;29:390–6.

137. Strong AL, Cederna PS, Rubin JP, et al. The current state of fat grafting: a review of harvesting, processing, and injection techniques. Plast Reconstr Surg 2015;136:897–912.

138. Coleman SR. Facial augmentation with structural fat grafting. Clin Plast Surg 2006;33:567–77.

139. Wang P, Wang Y, Zhang Z, et al. Comprehensive consideration and design with the virtual surgical planning-assisted treatment for hemifacial microsomia in adult patients. J Craniomaxillofac Surg 2018;46:1268–74.

140. Wang P, Zhang Z, Wang Y, et al. The accuracy of virtual-surgical-planning-assisted treatment of hemifacial microsomia in adult patients: distraction osteogenesis vs. orthognathic surgery. Int J Oral Maxillofac Surg 2018. https://doi.org/10.1016/j.ijom.2018.07.026.

141. Qin Z, Zhang Z, Li X, et al. One-Stage treatment for maxillofacial asymmetry with orthognathic and contouring surgery using virtual surgical planning and 3D-printed surgical templates. J Plast Reconstr Aesthet Surg 2018. https://doi.org/10.1016/j.bjps.2018.08.015.

142. Jaisinghani S, Adams NS, Mann RJ, et al. Virtual surgical planning in orthognathic surgery. Eplasty 2017;17:ic1.

143. Polley JW, Figueroa AA. Orthognathic positioning system: intraoperative system to transfer virtual surgical plan to operating field during orthognathic surgery. J Oral Maxillofac Surg 2013;71:911–20.

144. Luquetti DV, Brajcich MR, Stock NM, et al. Healthcare and psychosocial experiences of individuals with craniofacial microsomia: patient and caregivers perspectives. Int J Pediatr Otorhinolaryngol 2018;107:164–75.

145. Johns AL, Im DD, Lewin SL. Early familial experiences with microtia: psychosocial implications for pediatric providers. Clin Pediatr (Phila) 2018;57:775–82.

146. Hamilton KV, Ormond KE, Moscarello T, et al. Exploring the Medical and psychosocial concerns of adolescents and young adults with craniofacial microsomia: a qualitative study. Cleft Palate Craniofac J 2018;55:1430–9.

Porous Polyethylene Ear Reconstruction

Youssef Tahiri, MD, MSc, FRCSC*, John Reinisch, MD

KEYWORDS

- Ear reconstruction • Microtia • Porous polyethylene • Implant

KEY POINTS

- The use of a porous high-density polyethylene implant covered by a well-vascularized fascial flap, most commonly the temporoparietal fascia flap, is a good alternative for microtia reconstruction.
- This method of reconstruction allows ear reconstruction before a child enters school as well as eliminates some of the disadvantages inherent with the autologous costochondral cartilage ear reconstruction.
- Excellent outcomes with minimal morbidity can be obtained using this technique. It also provides a more holistic approach because it is done at a younger age, in a single stage, as an outpatient and could address the functional hearing issues earlier.

INTRODUCTION

The traditional surgical method of ear reconstruction involves the carving of a framework made from rib cartilage. Tanzer[1] described this technique almost 6 decades ago. Although Tanzer recommended ear reconstruction in the preschool period to minimize the "psychic trauma of a conspicuous deformity," the more recent modifications of Tanzer's framework have required harvesting a greater amount of costal cartilage. The age of ear reconstruction has thus been delayed from preschool years to age 10 years or older by many surgeons.[2–6] The psychological morbidity associated with an auricular deformity is well documented.[7] The need for more cartilage and the delay of treatment made costochondral ear reconstruction a more arduous physical and psychological endeavor for both children and their parents. Thus, if the final cosmetic result is not ideal, the entire reconstructive journey can be very disappointing.

An alternative method for ear reconstruction uses a polyethylene framework. The ability to reconstruct an ear before a child enters school is one of the major advantages of using an alloplastic framework. This method uses a porous high-density polyethylene (pHDPE) implant covered by a well-vascularized fascial flap, most commonly the superficial temporal parietal fascia (STPF) flap. This method of reconstruction eliminates some of the disadvantages inherent with the autologous costochondral cartilage ear reconstruction. It allows one to reconstruct reliably a realistic-appearing ear with minimal morbidity as well as a low rate of postoperative complications.

This article describes this technique that the senior author (J.R.) has been refining for over the past 28 years.

SURGICAL TECHNIQUE
Markings and Vascular Considerations

The superficial temporal artery (STA) system, along with its anterior and posterior branches, is identified either by palpation or via Doppler and is then marked. Often, the anterior branch of the STA runs just posteriorly to the frontal branch of

The authors have nothing to disclose.

Craniofacial and Pediatric Plastic Surgery, Cedars Sinai Medical Center, 250 N. Robertson Boulevard, Suite 506, Beverly Hills, CA, 90211

* Corresponding author.

E-mail address: Youssef_tahiri@hotmail.com

Clin Plastic Surg 46 (2019) 223–230

https://doi.org/10.1016/j.cps.2018.11.006

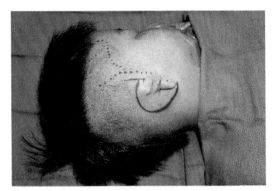

Fig. 1. The STA system, along with its anterior and posterior branches, is identified. The anterior branch of the STA runs just posteriorly to the frontal branch of the facial nerve.

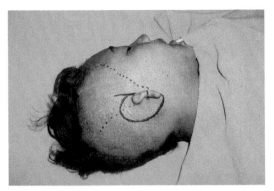

Fig. 3. The contralateral "normal" ear is outlined on a template and transposed onto the affected side.

the facial nerve (Fig. 1). At approximately 12 cm above the ear canal, this anterior branch runs transversely in a posterior direction (Fig. 2).

Following marking of the vascular system, the patient's contralateral "normal" ear is outlined on a template and transposed onto the affected side (Fig. 3). The STPF flap is then marked. It should be large enough to cover the implant without tension. The flap's width and height should be approximately 10 cm and 13 cm, respectively. The flap should include the transverse portion of the anterior branch of the STA (which could be a considered a superior landmark). The anterior

border of the flap is immediately anterior to the anterior branch of the STA (Fig. 4).

In some instances, the STA has an origin posterior to the lobule and runs right under the microtic cartilage. It is important to be mindful of this anatomic variation (Fig. 5). Resection of the microtic cartilage has to be performed with care to prevent injury of the STA.

Finally, the lobule is marked for posterior transposition (Fig. 6).

Superficial Temporoparietal Fascia Flap Harvest

Following anterior reflection of the ear remnant and mastoid skin, the scalp is elevated from the

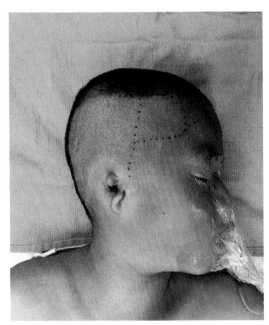

Fig. 2. At approximately 12 cm above the ear canal, this anterior branch runs transversely in a posterior direction.

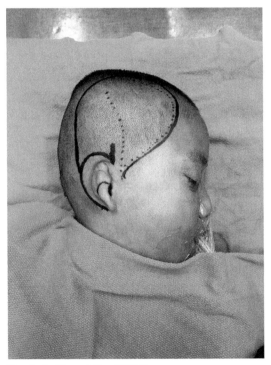

Fig. 4. Outline of the STPE flap.

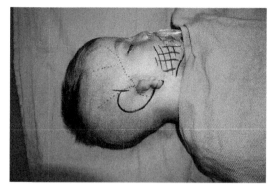

Fig. 5. In approximately 20% of the cases, the STA has an origin posterior to the lobule and runs right under the microtic cartilage. In these instances, resection of the microtic cartilage has to be performed with care to prevent injury of the STA.

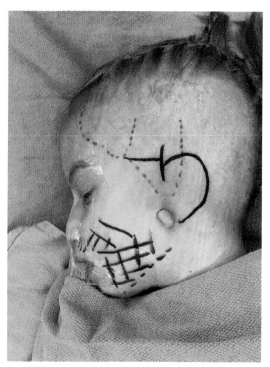

Fig. 7. The original incision can be extended horizontally across the upper sideburn if necessary to facilitate dissection.

surface of the STPF. The proper dissection plane is at the junction of the fascia and subcutaneous fat layer. The dissection is carried using a blended cautery using the "cut" function (not "coag"). It is of prime importance to stay superficial enough to not injure the STA and its branches while staying deep enough to not injure hair follicles. A horizontal extension of the incision across the upper sideburn can be added if necessary to facilitate dissection (**Fig. 7**).

Once the scalp elevation is complete, an incision through the superficial temporal fascia and underlying subgaleal fascia is made down to the deep temporal fascia immediately anterior to the anterior branch of the STA. The posterior border of the STPF flap is also incised and carried through the subgaleal fascia to the periosteum. Through the upper portion of this posterior incision, the upper scalp (cephalic to the scalp elevation) is dissected bluntly in the subgaleal space with a no. 22 urethral sound. The sound can be tunneled

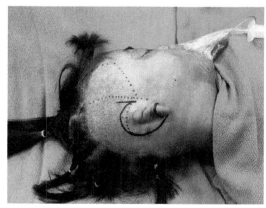

Fig. 6. The lobule is marked for posterior transposition.

above the periosteum and to elevate the scalp from the periosteum 3 to 4 cm beyond the 13-cm upper border of the scalp dissection on top of the STSP fascia. This blunt elevation of the scalp facilitates the eventual division of the distal cephalic border of the STPF flap from the undersurface of the scalp.

The STPE is then converted into an inferiorly based flap along with its subgaleal layer, by dividing these 2 layers from the undersurface of the scalp superiorly with a long, angled Colorado tip needle (Stryker, Kalamazoo, MI, USA). The STPF and its underlying subgaleal layer are then bluntly dissected from the periosteum superiorly and the deep temporal fascia inferiorly. It is important to include the thin subgaleal areolar fascia with the STPF flap. This loose areolar layer becomes the outer surface of the temporal parietal fascia (TPF) flap upon which the skin is placed. This layer allows the healed skin graft to move over the STPF, which becomes adherent to the porous implant. The inferiorly based superficial temporal fascia is then transposed inferiorly through the mastoid opening (**Fig. 8**).

Implant Insetting and Coverage

To prevent postoperative caudal descent of the implant, a 1-cm-wide, inferiorly based, vertically

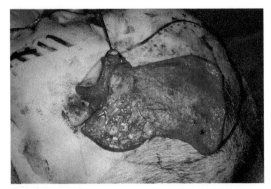

Fig. 8. The inferiorly based STPE flap is transposed inferiorly through the mastoid opening. The base flap should start a few centimeters below the future site of the helical rim to allow for a good sulcus between the scalp and the reconstructed ear.

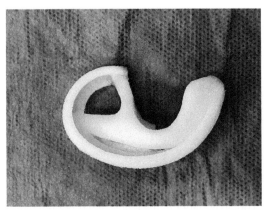

Fig. 10. The implant consists of a base and a helical rim. The base component is carved by removing the tragal component. The helical root is removed to create a larger conchal bowl. The helical rim is attached to the base, using remnants of polyethylene material from the removed helical root or tragal extension. The 2 pieces are melted together with a battery-operated, high-temperature ophthalmic cautery.

oriented flap of deep temporal fascia can be raised from the temporalis muscle to suspend the implant. This narrow flap must be tunneled through the base of STPF flap using a very fine-tip pediatric hemostat. To avoid injury to the vascular pedicle, the flap should be transilluminated to identify the vascular pedicle when making the tunnel (**Fig. 9**).

The custom-made implant (**Fig. 10**) is then positioned in its appropriate location. The leash is wrapped around the anterior portion of the inferior crus of the ear implant and sutured to itself.

One suction drain is then placed beneath the implant, and another one is placed under the scalp, where the flap was harvested. Both drains exit through the parietal scalp, posterior to the ear.

The auricular implant is then completely covered by the fascia flap, and skrink-wrapping of the fascia is observed once suction is applied (**Fig. 11**).

A full-thickness skin graft from the groin is used to cover the posterior aspect of the ear. The

anterior and lateral aspect of the ear is usually covered by the non-hair-bearing residual microtic and mastoid skin. This skin can be used as an anteriorly based flap or as a full-thickness skin graft (**Fig. 12**). When additional skin is required, a full-thickness skin graft from the contralateral postauricular skin is used. In the case of bilateral microtia, the anterior/lateral surface of the ear can be covered using a full-thickness skin graft from the inner upper arm or supraclavicular area, because the contralateral post-auricular skin is not an option.

Tragal Reconstruction

Tragal reconstruction involves the placement of an appropriately sized piece of cartilage from the

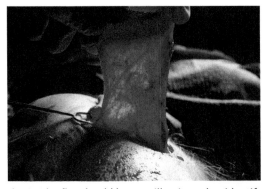

Fig. 9. The flap should be transilluminated to identify the vascular pedicle when making the tunnel for the suspending leash to avoid injury to the vascular pedicle.

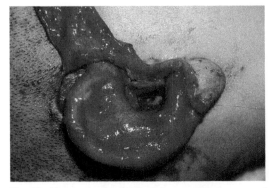

Fig. 11. The auricular implant is completely covered by the fascia, and skrink-wrapping of the fascia is observed once suction is applied.

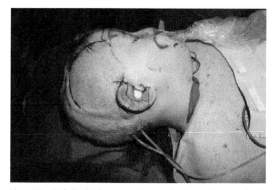

Fig. 12. A full-thickness skin graft from the groin is used to cover the posterior aspect of the ear. The anterior and lateral aspect of the ear is usually covered by the non-hair-bearing residual microtic and mastoid skin. This skin can be used as an anteriorly based flap or as a full-thickness skin graft. If more skin is needed, it is harvested from the contralateral postauricular area (if unilateral microtia) or from the contralateral inner upper arm (if bilateral microtia).

resected cartilage remnant into a preauricular pocket. This pocket is created by medial transposition of an anteriorly based horizontally oriented flap of skin. Once positioned correctly, the cartilage is fixated using a 5-0 chromic gut mattress suture (**Fig. 13**).

Dressing and Postoperative Care

Once the reconstruction is complete, the ear is then covered with an antibiotic ointment, and an alginate dressing is placed into the conchal bowl and along the postauricular sulcus. A custom-made silicone ear splint is then fabricated and

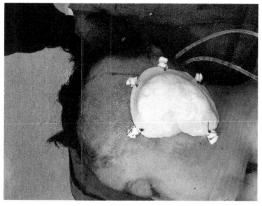

Fig. 14. A custom-made silicone ear splint is then fabricated and applied to the ear. It is contoured to the ear and allowed to become firm before being sutured to the surrounding scalp and cheek with horizontal mattress sutures of 2-0 Prolene tied over silicone pledgets.

applied to the ear. It is contoured to the ear and allowed to become firm before being sutured to the surrounding scalp and cheek with horizontal mattress sutures of 2-0 Prolene tied over silicone pledgets (**Fig. 14**). The head is then wrapped with an absorptive head dressing after the drains are removed, and a decorative head cap is applied to the dressing (**Fig. 15**).

On the second day after surgery, the absorptive dressing is removed, whereas the protective silicone mold stays in place for a total of 2 weeks. Two weeks following surgery, the mold is removed and the ear is washed and cleaned. A new mold is fabricated. It will be worn only at night over the next 4 months. It will help maintain an adequate posterior sulcus.

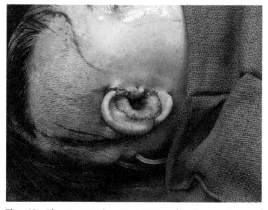

Fig. 13. The tragus is reconstructed using a piece of resected microtic cartilage remnant and inserting it into a preauricular pocket created by medial transposition of an anteriorly based horizontally oriented flap of skin.

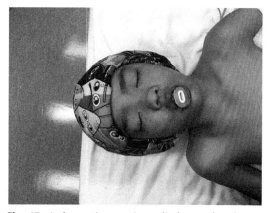

Fig. 15. A decorative cap is applied over the absorptive dressing. The patient will keep this dressing on for 2 days. On the second day after surgery, the absorptive dressing is removed, whereas the protective silicone mold stays in place for a total of 2 weeks.

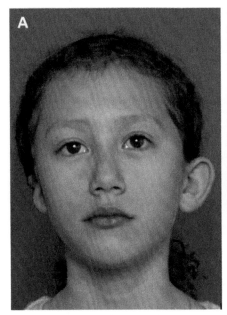 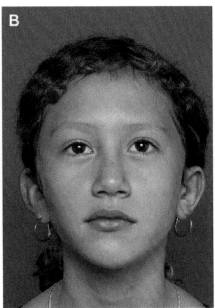

Fig. 16. (*A*) A 7-year-old girl with right-sided microtia. (*B*) She successfully underwent pHDPE ear reconstruction. This is her 2-year follow-up.

Figs. 16–18 depict 3 patients who underwent successfully pHDPE ear reconstruction.

DISCUSSION

The use of an alloplastic framework is an alternative approach to ear reconstruction. The senior author (J.R.) developed the procedure over a 28-year period and has performed more than 1500 ear reconstructions using a polyethylene implant covered by either a temporal-parietal or an occipital-parietal facial flap. This large experience with extensive follow-up has allowed modifications to improve outcomes and reduce complications. It is clear that polyethylene ear framework can provide an excellent and long-lasting ear reconstruction. However, it is important to understand the differences between an autologous cartilage framework and a polyethylene ear framework.

Both cartilage and polyethylene frameworks are passive skeletons that provide shape and projection to the covering soft tissue. Cartilage has a low metabolic requirement because it has relatively few active cells within a large extracellular matrix. As a result, it survives nicely as a graft and is well tolerated beneath a thin skin flap. By contrast, when a porous polyethylene implant is placed beneath a thin skin flap, a significant rate of exposure of the implant is seen over time. A polyethylene implant should never be substituted for a cartilage framework when performing the traditional mastoid skin pocket soft tissue coverage.

A polyethylene framework requires a different type of soft tissue coverage to avoid exposures. Early in his series, the senior author (J.R.) learned that covering the entire alloplastic material with a temporal-parietal or occipital-parietal fascia flap reduces exposures to a very low rate (<4%). The covering fascia must be well vascularized, must include its underlying loose areolar layer, and must be large enough to envelope the entire implant without tension.[8] With cartilage reconstruction, the harvest and assembly of the framework are the most time-consuming aspects of the procedure. With an alloplastic reconstruction, the soft tissue coverage of the framework becomes the largest and most critical component of the surgery. Adequate color-matched full-thickness skin grafts are then placed over the turned over fascial flap.

In the rare instances whereby the TPF has been used or damaged, an implant can be still covered by an occipital flap based on the occipital artery and can allow an adequate and successful ear reconstruction.

The authors prefer to use a porous polyethylene ear reconstruction because, in their experience, it better addresses the cosmetic, functional, and psychological issues associated with microtia (**Box 1**). Although surgeons have modified Tanzer's technique of ear reconstruction to reduce the number of required operative stages,[1,3–6]

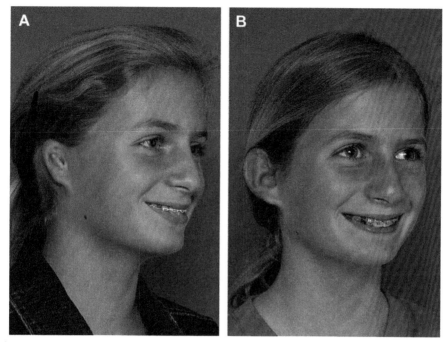

Fig. 17. (*A*) A 12-year-old girl with right-sided microtia. (*B*) She successfully underwent pHDPE ear reconstruction. This is her 1-year follow-up.

these refinements require a larger amount of costal cartilage. To be able to obtain a greater amount of cartilage, surgeons have postponed the age of ear reconstruction from the age originally recommended by Tanzer to 10 years and older. This delay in the age of reconstruction with autologous cartilage is both psychologically and socially difficult for children and their family.

The use of an alloplastic framework allows ear reconstruction before children start school and are exposed to potential peer ridicule. Early ear reconstruction is possible because the growth of

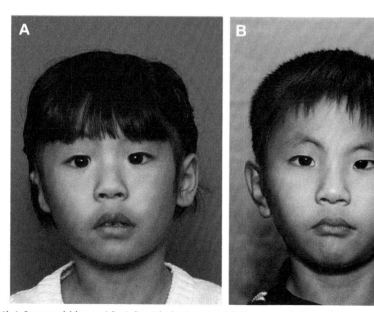

Fig. 18. (*A*) A 3-year-old boy with right-sided microtia. (*B*) He successfully underwent pHDPE ear reconstruction. This is his 2.5-year follow-up.

Box 1
Advantages of ear reconstruction with a porous high-density polyethylene implant covered by a well-vascularized fascia flap

Ear reconstruction performed before entering school

Early atresia repair can be performed before or at the same time as external ear reconstruction

Outpatient procedure

Single-stage procedure

Minimal morbidity

Accurate placement and better symmetry in patients with facial asymmetry (such as hemifacial microsomia or Treacher Collins syndrome) or low hairline

the normal ear reaches 85% of adult size by 3.5 years.[9] The use of a large fascia flap provides sufficient soft tissue coverage so that the reconstructed ear can match the projection of the opposite ear, and therefore, can be done as a single-stage surgery. By eliminating the costal cartilage harvest, the surgery produces minimal discomfort and can be done as an outpatient with its obvious psychological and economic advantages.

The functional component of ear reconstruction has often been ignored by plastic surgeons. Hearing loss is an important issue associated with microtia. Although normal hearing from the opposite ear in unilateral microtia might allow acquisition of speech, there are several issues with unilateral hearing loss (sound localization, difficulty hearing in noise, lack of binaural summation, compromised language acquisition) that become more evident in older children and adults. Furthermore, emerging data supporting amblyaudia as a diagnostic entity highlight the importance of early hearing management.[10] Amblyaudia is a term used to describe persistent hearing difficulty experienced by individuals with a history of asymmetric hearing loss during a critical early window of brain development.

To avoid damaging the virgin mastoid skin needed to cover a cartilage framework, an atresia repair is generally performed after the costal cartilage framework is placed. On the other hand, because an alloplastic framework must be covered by transposition of an adjacent arterial fascia flap, the tissue needed to cover the alloplastic framework is not jeopardized by a prior, early canalplasty. Thus, an atresia repair can be performed before or even at the same time as an alloplastic ear reconstruction.

Furthermore, autologous ear reconstruction requires healthy and ideally non-hair-bearing skin

flaps, making the reconstruction more challenging in patients with very low hairlines (seen, for example, in Treacher Collins patients) or with traumatized/scared auricular/temporal cutaneous area. This is not the case in alloplastic ear reconstruction, because the framework's coverage does not rely on the native mastoid skin, but on the fascial flap and skin grafts. The ear is thus placed at the appropriate position irrespective of the hairline or previous scars.

SUMMARY

To conclude, the use of a pHDPE implant covered with a well-vascularized fascial flap allows one to obtain excellent ear reconstruction outcomes with minimal morbidity. This technique provides a more holistic approach because it is done at a younger age, in a single stage, as an outpatient and could address the functional hearing issues earlier.

REFERENCES

1. Tanzer RC. Total reconstruction of the external ear. Plast Reconstr Surg Transplant Bull 1959;23(1):1–15.
2. Wallace CG, Mao HY, Wang CJ, et al. Three- dimensional computed tomography reveals different donor-site deformities in adult and growing microtia patients despite total subperichondrial costal cartilage harvest and donor-site recon- struction. Plast Reconstr Surg 2014;133(3):640–51.
3. Brent B. The correction of microtia with autgenous cartilage grafts:1. The classic deformity? Plast Reconstr Surg 1980;66(1):1–12.
4. Nagata S, Fukuda O. A new reconstruction for the lobule type microtia. Jpn J Plast Reconstr Surg 1987;7:689.
5. Firmin F. Ear reconstruction in cases of typical microtia: personal experience based on 352 microtic ear corrections. Scand J Plast Reconstr Surg Hand Surg 1998;32(1):35–47.
6. Ksrai L, Snyder-Warwick A, Fisher D. Single-stage autologous ear reconstruction for microtia. Plast Reconstr Surg 2014;133(3):652–62.
7. Horlock N, Vögelin E, Bradbury ET, et al. Psychosocial outcome of patients after ear reconstruction: a retrospective study of 62 patients. Ann Plast Surg 2005;54:517–24.
8. Reinisch J. Ear reconstruction in young children. Facial Plast Surg 2015;31(6):600–3.
9. Adamson J, Horton C, Crawford H. The growth pattern of the external ear. Plast Reconstr Surg 1965;36(4):466–70.
10. Kaplan AB, Kozin ED, Remenschneider A, et al. Amblyaudia: review of pathophysiology, clinical presentation, and treatment of a new diagnosis. Otolaryngol Head Neck Surg 2016;154(2):247–55.

Parry Romberg Syndrome

Kelly P. Schultz, BA, Elaine Dong, BA, Tuan A. Truong, MD,
Renata S. Maricevich, MD*

KEYWORDS

- Parry-Romberg syndrome • Progressive hemifacial atrophy • Microsurgical reconstruction

KEY POINTS

- Parry-Romberg syndrome is a rare disease characterized by unilateral facial soft tissue atrophy that may progress to involve underlying structures.
- Extracutaneous disease manifestations are common and require an interdisciplinary management approach.
- Reconstruction of hemifacial atrophy in patients with Parry-Romberg syndrome is a surgical challenge.
- Commonly used techniques include synthetic injections, autologous fat grafting, orthognathic surgery, and microsurgical reconstruction.

INTRODUCTION

Parry-Romberg syndrome (PRS) is a rare craniofacial disorder characterized by hemifacial atrophy of the skin, subcutaneous tissue, fat, and, in severe cases, underlying muscle and bone. Disease onset is typically within the first 20 years of life, although cases of later onset have been described.[1] Symptoms progress over a 2- to 10-year self-limited period before spontaneous stabilization.[2–4] Extracutaneous disease manifestations, including neurologic, ocular, and oral pathology, are common and may present at any stage of disease.[1]

The current literature best describes PRS as mild, moderate, or severe, to stratify disease and guide patient management.[5]

- Mild disease is described as skin and subcutaneous tissue atrophy limited to a single sensory branch of the trigeminal nerve.
- Moderate disease is described as atrophy limited to 2 branches of the trigeminal nerve.
- Severe disease is described as atrophy in a distribution involving all 3 branches of the trigeminal nerve or any bone involvement (**Fig. 1**).

PATHOGENESIS

The pathogenesis of PRS remains unknown, although various mechanisms of disease have been proposed and debated.[6] PRS is most often described as an autoimmune condition on the same spectrum of disease as localized scleroderma *en coupe de sabre*, a variant of localized scleroderma involving the frontoparietal face and skull.[7] This pattern is supported by findings of inflammatory histopathology, serum autoantibodies, coexistent autoimmune diseases (eg, lupus), and positive response to immunosuppression in patients with PRS.[1]

Neurologically based theories suggest that PRS may be the result of disordered developmental migration of neural crest cells, neurotrophic viral infection, trigeminal peripheral neuritis,[5] intracranial vascular malformation,[8] or peripheral sympathetic nervous system dysfunction after traumatic disruption of the cervical plexus or thoracic sympathetic trunk.[3]

Disclosure Statement: The authors have nothing to disclose.
Division of Plastic Surgery, Baylor College of Medicine, 6701 Fannin Street, Houston, TX 77030
* Corresponding author. Division of Plastic Surgery, Michael E. DeBakey Department of Surgery, Baylor College of Medicine, 6701 Fannin Street, Suite 610.00, Houston, TX 77030.
E-mail address: renata.maricevich@bcm.edu

Clin Plastic Surg 46 (2019) 231–237
https://doi.org/10.1016/j.cps.2018.11.007

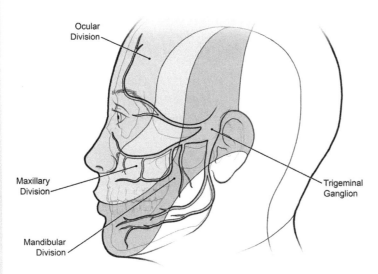

Fig. 1. Distribution of first (ocular), second (maxillary), and third (mandibular) branches of the trigeminal nerve. In classification of Parry-Romberg syndrome, mild disease is characterized by skin and subcutaneous atrophy in 1 sensory branch of the trigeminal nerve, moderate disease is characterized by atrophy in 2 branches, and severe disease may be characterized by atrophy in all 3 branches or any bone involvement.

PRESENTATION AND EVALUATION
Disease Presentation

Skin and soft tissue involvement

PRS characteristically manifests on the face, caudal to the forehead.[4] Atrophy begins superficially, although the epidermis is minimally affected, and may progress to involve the subcutaneous tissue, fat, fascia, muscle, cartilage, and bone.[2,9] Alopecia and hyperpigmentation or depigmentation are commonly seen overlying the atrophic tissue.[1] Nearly all cases involve the cheek, periorbital and perioral areas; more progressive cases may spread to involve the nasolabial fold, brow, ear, and neck.[2]

Neurologic involvement

PRS has been described as a neurocutaneous syndrome, because the most common systemic disease manifestations are neurologically based.[3] Seizures, migraines, hemiplegia, aneurysms, brain atrophy, cranial neuropathies (cranial nerves III, V, VI, and VII), intracranial vascular malformations, trigeminal neuralgia, cognitive impairment, and behavioral disorders have been reported in association with PRS.[1,5]

Ophthalmologic involvement

The most commonly reported ocular finding is enophthalmos secondary to orbital, malar, and maxillary subcutaneous tissue deficiency. Other ophthalmologic manifestations include ophthalmoplegia, strabismus, iris heterochromia, and uveitis.[2] Patients with neurologic symptoms may experience optic nerve dysfunction, neuroretinopathy, or Horner syndrome.[5] In cases of eyelid soft tissue atrophy and retraction, exposure keratopathy is a concern, and intervention is critical to prevent permanent corneal scarring and preserve vision.[1]

Oral involvement

PRS with oral cavity involvement most frequently affects the tongue, gingiva, and soft palate. Delayed tooth eruption and dental root exposure or resorption are relatively common, whereas more extensive tooth or mandibular atrophy may be seen in severe cases (**Fig. 2**). Temporomandibular joint involvement often manifests as pain with mastication and difficulty or complete inability to open the mouth or perform normal jaw movements.[1]

Clinical Evaluation and Diagnosis

PRS is a largely clinical diagnosis, but no universal diagnostic criteria currently exist. Effective evaluation of patients with suspected PRS involves 4 major elements: a complete disease history, a physical examination with attention to the head and neck, consideration of potential differential diagnoses, and attention to the patient's psychological health. A careful history should reveal progressive symptom onset and any systemic disease manifestations.[10] Examination should pay careful attention to facial asymmetry, particularly in the maxillary, malar, and orbital regions.[2]

PRS may be difficult to differentiate from localized scleroderma *en coupe de sabre* on initial evaluation, because both conditions have a similar age of onset and progressive course. Generally, a diagnosis of PRS should be made in cases of widespread unilateral soft tissue atrophy with thin or soft overlying skin that is not preceded by

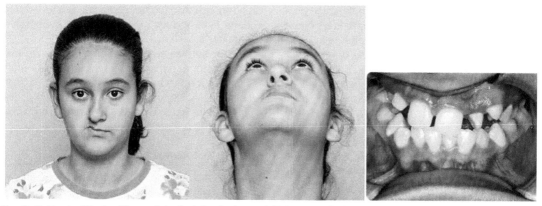

Fig. 2. Patient with significant right facial soft tissue deficiency, with dental and skeletal changes.

inflammation or induration. localized scleroderma *en coupe de sabre* presents with cutaneous sclerosis localized to the frontoparietal region involving the forehead.[3,11] In addition, referral to a rheumatologist may help to differentiate other similar soft tissue connective disorders.

The importance of screening for psychological or relational disorders cannot be overstated. Patients often suffer significant loss of self-confidence after the progression of soft tissue deficiency, and may be discouraged if presenting after failure of multiple treatments.[5] Preoperative and postoperative psychiatric consultations should be offered.

Additional Workup

After a diagnosis of PRS, further steps are necessary to ascertain the severity of disease and to guide appropriate management strategies. Computed tomography scanning is indicated in most cases to assess or confirm bone hypotrophy. MRI is the study of choice in the evaluation of neurologic symptoms and often reveals white matter hyperintense signaling ipsilateral to soft tissue involvement. Lumbar puncture and electroencephalography are only indicated for seizure workup. Doppler ultrasound studies may be beneficial in the detection of possible arteriovenous malformation in areas of significant soft tissue atrophy.[5] Even with a low suspicion for ocular involvement, ophthalmology consultation is necessary to properly evaluate the patient's visual acuity, extraocular movements, intraocular pressure, and optic disc to prevent eventual visual impairment.[4]

Laboratory studies are unrevealing in PRS diagnosis and workup. Many patients have positive serum antinuclear antibodies and some may have elevated rheumatoid factor or anticardiolipin antibodies, but these findings are nonspecific and have no role in disease management.[4]

TREATMENT
Disease Management

Management of PRS involves stabilization of systemic symptoms and aesthetic improvement of soft tissue deficiency. This process should begin with noninvasive medical management at the time of diagnosis to prevent further disease progression. Although the condition's unclear etiology prevents curative or targeted medical therapy, there are reports of limited success with trials of D-penicillamine, oral steroids, methotrexate, antimalarial medications, retinoids, topical steroids, and vitamin D analogs plus Photochemotherapy with Psoralens and long wave ultraviolet radiation.[12] Interdisciplinary management is critical in cases of neurologic, ophthalmologic, cardiac, or other major system involvement.

The major aesthetic challenge and goal of treatment for patients with PRS is the restoration of facial contour and symmetry. There is controversy regarding the ideal timing of reconstructive intervention. The current literature broadly suggests proceeding after a 1- to 2-year period of stable disease, but this recommendation changes with disease extent and desired procedure.

Reconstruction often begins with autologous or synthetic fillers and continues with increasingly invasive procedures as indicated for the extent of tissue involvement. Surgical options include fat grafting, orthognathic surgery, and free tissue transfer, with most patients requiring a combination of various techniques.

Synthetic Tissue Fillers

Synthetic tissue fillers are the least invasive option for the correction of facial contour defects, with the advantage of requiring only a single-stage procedure. Injectable calcium hydroxyapatite, poly-L-lactic acid, silicone, and polyethylene have been used in successful correction of mild or moderate soft tissue atrophy.[5,13] Feldman and colleagues[14] have recently reported successful correction of enophthalmos, lagophthalmos, and exposure keratopathy with hyaluronic acid injectables.

Limitations of synthetic tissue fillers include postprocedure resorption and foreign body reaction.[5] Consistent reapplication, although costly, is required to maintain optimal facial contour. Foreign body reactions may involve inflammation, ulceration, or thrombosis at the injection site.[15] To date, no foreign material has proven to be completely safe, stable, nondegradable, and diffusion or migration resistant. Fat grafting is often preferred over synthetic injectables because the procedure carries a lower risk of infection, seroma, scarring, and migration.[13]

Autologous Fat Grafting

Autologous fat grafting, or lipoinjection, has been shown to provide exceptional soft tissue restoration in patients with PRS. It is readily available, relatively inexpensive, and may be harvested repeatedly.[16] The Coleman technique, also known as structural fat grafting or LipoStructure, is most commonly used and involves the purification of harvested fat via centrifugation and reinjection of fat in small aliquots to ensure proper proximity to a vascular supply.[17] When performed in stages, deep compartments are grafted first to establish proper tissue projection, and subsequent sessions focus on superficial compartments to perfect facial contour.[18] (Fig. 3) Serial injections alone may be sufficient for patients with mild or moderate disease, whereas patients with severe disease often undergo fat grafting in conjunction with other operations. In these cases, lipoinjection at the time of free tissue transfer creates a more seamless transition between the host and transplanted tissue in the immediate postoperative period, often necessitating fewer flap revision operations.[19]

Grafted fat tissue undoubtedly undergoes some degree of postprocedure resorption and hypertrophies if postoperative weight gain occurs. Patients with PRS, especially those who have undergone previous craniofacial bone surgery, have even poorer graft retention than the general population (41% vs 80%).[13,18,20] Most volume resorption will be apparent at the 3-month postprocedure evaluation, at which time subsequent lipoinjections may be performed if there are no signs of residual postoperative inflammation. Overcorrection of facial asymmetry in initial procedures is often recommended to compensate for postoperative volume loss and limit the number of successive injections.[18]

Recent studies suggest addition of insulin-like growth factor and platelet-rich plasma to the graft maximizes long-term outcomes and reduces graft resorption. In the future, concurrent adipose-derived stem cell transplant may better enhance retention.[18]

Skeletal Reconstruction

Patients who develop PRS early, before puberty or even as early as preschool age, are at a higher risk of facial skeleton deformities. Hypoplasia of the maxilla, mandible, zygoma, temporal bone, and frontal bone are commonly seen.[21] Reconstructive options include orthognathic surgery, bone or cartilage grafting, and implant augmentation.

Patients with significant deviation of the maxilla and mandible will require orthognathic surgery before soft tissue transfer to establish a stable skeletal foundation and optimal occlusion.[9,20] A Le Fort I osteotomy with subsequent autogenous bone grafting to fill the remaining bone gap is often performed in a single stage. In more severe cases, mandibular lengthening may be indicated with second-stage Le Fort I or sagittal split osteotomy 6 to 8 months later. If indicated, osseous genioplasty, in isolation or at the time of orthognathic surgery, is performed to correct abnormalities or atrophy of the chin prominence.[21,22]

Onlay bone graft, with harvest from the rib or calvarium, may be used at the time of free tissue flap to correct atrophy of the zygoma or maxillary buttress; however, some degree of postoperative resorption is expected with the use of nonvascularized bone or cartilage grafts.[23,24] Alternatively, porous polyethylene implants may be used in reconstruction of the zygoma, maxilla, chin prominence, and mandible, because they are malleable and provide an optimal foundation for vascular and soft tissue ingrowth.[21]

Free Tissue Transplantation

Free tissue transfer is the gold standard for large-volume reconstruction in patients with severe soft tissue atrophy, providing superior long-term functional and aesthetic results to previously mentioned methods.[5,19] Satisfactory aesthetic outcomes have been described with the use of various free flaps, including the greater omentum, groin, latissimus dorsi, parascapular, dorsal thoracic, and anterolateral thigh. Advantages and disadvantages of each flap should be considered. The ideal free flap material for facial soft tissue repair should have a texture similar to that of the

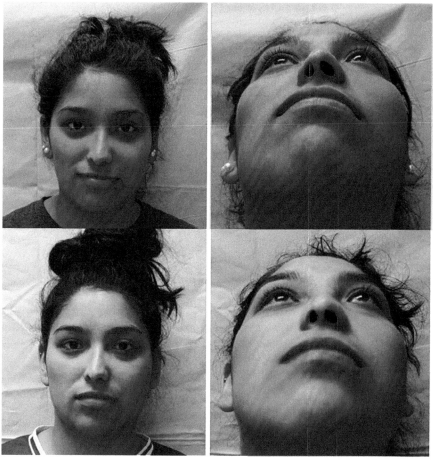

Fig. 3. Patient with right side soft tissue deficiency preoperative and postoperative first round of fat grafting.

subcutaneous tissue, be able to conform to the defect, and undergo minimal postoperative growth or migration.[23]

Greater omental free flaps were commonly used at the arrival of microsurgery; however, they are particularly susceptible to postoperative sagging owing to a lack of inherent structural strength and are not routinely used.[5]

Groin free flap transplantation was previously the most commonly used technique in microsurgical reconstruction of PRS-related soft tissue defects, according to Agostini and colleagues.[16] The major advantage that groin flaps offer is a relatively unnoticeable donor site defect[25]; however, this advantage is offset by the significant susceptibility to graft volume increase with postoperative patient growth and weight gain, almost always requiring staged revision.[5,23]

Latissimus dorsi free flap offers excellent compliance, a long vascular pedicle, abundant tissue, hairless skin, and minimal sagging relative to other donor sites. Reported disadvantages include

poor facial skin color match and a conspicuous donor site scar.[5] In addition, the flap is not amenable to fine contour modification with liposuction.

The parascapular flap, based on the descending cutaneous branch of the circumflex scapular artery, also has a long vascular pedicle, exceptional structural strength, abundant and compact subcutaneous fat, and a thick dermis.[5] The dorsal thoracic adipofascial free flap, also referred to as the circumflex scapular artery-based adipofascial flap, includes the fascial components of both scapular and parascapular fasciocutanous flaps, providing thin but large dimension coverage. Advantages of this flap include less donor site damage and scapular scarring in comparison with the scapular or parascapular flap.[19]

The anterolateral thigh flap offers a large soft tissue volume, large vascular pedicle, and minimal donor site morbidity; however, the flap's substantial weight confers a large risk of postoperative ptosis. Significant fatty tissue removal with preservation of the dermis and subdermal plexus should be performed to thin the flap appropriately before implantation.[26]

The proper timing of microvascular surgery is highly debated. Many surgeons prefer to defer surgery until the disease has completely stabilized; however, there are reports that free tissue transfer effectively inhibits or slows down disease progression when performed in cases of active disease.[16] Initiation of treatment before disease burn-out is also associated with an increased number of total procedures but improved overall patient satisfaction and a presumed reduction in potential psychosocial harm.[22]

Extensive preoperative planning is imperative for all microsurgical procedures. The design of an appropriate flap for facial contour correction, while accounting for flap shrinkage after harvest, is a technically challenging process. Current literature describes use of facial plaster templates or, more recently, creation of a facial profile with 3-dimensional laser scanning systems to assist flap construction.[19,26]

Free flap transfer, as the most invasive of current PRS management options, carries the greatest risk of hematoma and infection. Other postoperative complications include partial flap loss, excess bulk, atrophy, dehiscence, seroma, and transient facial nerve palsy. The majority of free tissue transfer procedures invariably require revision surgeries for flap thinning or resuspension.[16]

SUMMARY

PRS is a rare craniofacial disorder that has been widely described in the literature. Although the pathogenesis of this disease is not currently known, many treatment options are available that may limit disease progression and provide patients with both functional and aesthetic improvement. Surgical management often involves a combination of synthetic filler injection, fat grafting, orthognathic surgery, and free tissue transplantation depending on the severity of disease. Free flap transfer remains the gold standard in augmentation of extensive soft tissue atrophy.

REFERENCES

1. Bucher F, Fricke J, Neugebauer A, et al. Ophthalmological manifestations of Parry-Romberg syndrome. Surv Ophthalmol 2016;61:693–701.
2. Buonaccorsi S, Leonardi A, Cavelli E, et al. Parry-Romberg syndrome. J Craniofac Surg 2005;16(6):1132–5.
3. El-Kehdy J, Abbas O, Rubeiz N. A review of Parry-Romberg syndrome. J Am Acad Dermatol 2012; 67:769–84.
4. Tolkachjov SN, Patel NG, Tollefson MM. Progressive hemifacial atrophy: a review. Orphanet J Rare Dis 2015;10:39.
5. Vaienti L, Soresina M, Menozzi A. Parascapular free flap and fat grafts: combined surgical methods in morphological restoration of hemifacial progressive atrophy. Plast Reconstr Surg 2005; 116:699–711.
6. Pensler JM, Murphy GF. Clinical and ultrastructural studies of Romberg's hemifacial atrophy. Plast Reconstr Surg 1990;85:669–76.
7. Garcia-de la Torre I, Castello-Sendra J, Esgleyes-Ribot T, et al. Autoantibodies in Parry Romberg syndrome: a serologic study of 14 patients. J Rheumatol 1995;22(1):73–7.
8. Pichiecchio A, Uggetti C, Grazia Egitto M, et al. Parry-Romberg syndrome with migraine and intracranial aneurysm. Neurology 2002;59:606.
9. Wojcicki P, Zachara M. Surgical treatment of patients with Parry-Romberg syndrome. Ann Plast Surg 2001;66:267–72.
10. Hunstad JP, Shifrin DA, Kortesis BG. Successful treatment of Parry-Romberg syndrome with autologous fat grafting: 14 year follow-up and review. Ann Plast Surg 2001;67:423–5.
11. Duymaz A, Karabekmez FE, Keskin M, et al. Parry-Romberg syndrome: facial atrophy and its relationship with other regions of the body. Ann Plast Surg 2009;63:457–61.
12. Tollefson MM, Witman PM. En coup de sabre morphea and Parry-Romberg syndrome: a retrospective review of 54 patients. J Am Acad Dermatol 2007;56: 257–63.
13. Ortega V, Sastoque D. New and successful technique for the management of Parry-Romberg syndrome's soft tissue atrophy. J Craniofac Surg 2015; 26:e507–10.
14. Feldman I, Sheptulin VA, Grusha YO, et al. Deep orbital sub-q hyaluronic acid filler injection for enophthalmic sighted eyes in parry-romberg syndrome. Ophthal Plast Reconstr Surg 2018. https://doi.org/10.1097/IOP.0000000000001050.
15. Szczerkowska-Dobosz A, Olszewska B, Lemanska M, et al. Acquired facial lipoatrophy: pathogenesis and therapeutic options. Postepy Dermatol Alergol 2015; 32:127–33.
16. Agostini T, Spinelli G, Marino G, et al. Esthetic restoration in progressive hemifacial atrophy (romberg disease): structural fat grafting versus local/free flaps. J Craniofac Surg 2014;25:783–7.
17. Coleman SR, Katzel EB. Fat grafting for facial filling and regeneration. Clin Plast Surg 2015;42: 289–300.
18. Denadai R, Raposo-Amaral CA, Pinho AS, et al. Predictors of autologous free fat graft retention in the management of craniofacial contour deformities. Plast Reconstr Surg 2017;140:50e–61e.

19. Song B, Li Y, Wang B, et al. Treatment of severe hemifacial atrophy with dorsal thoracic adipofascial freeflap and concurrent lipoinjection. J Craniofac Surg 2015;26:e162–6.

20. Slack GC, Tabit CJ, Allam KA, et al. Parry-Romberg reconstruction: beneficial results despite poorer fat take. Ann Plast Surg 2014;73:307–10.

21. Hu J, Yin L, Tang X, et al. Combined skeletal and soft tissue reconstruction for severe Parry-Romberg syndrome. J Craniofac Surg 2011;23:937–41.

22. Slack GC, Tabit CJ, Allam KA, et al. Parry-Romberg reconstruction: optimal timing for hard and soft tissue procedures. J Craniofac Surg 2012;23:1969–73.

23. Baek R, Heo C, Kim BK. Use of various free flaps in progressive hemifacial atrophy. J Craniofac Surg 2011;22:2268–71.

24. Myung Y, Lee YH, Chang H. Surgical correction of progressive hemifacial atrophy with onlay bone graft combined with soft tissue augmentation. J Craniofac Surg 2012;23:1841–4.

25. Dunkley MP, Stevenson JH. Experience with the free "inverted" groin flap in facial and soft tissue contouring: a report on 6 flaps. Br J Plast Surg 1990;43:154.

26. Chai G, Tan A, Yao C, et al. Treating Parry Romberg syndrome using three-dimensional scanning and printing and the anterolateral thigh dermal adipofascial flap. J Craniofac Surg 2015;26:1826–9.

Pediatric Facial Trauma

Tom W. Andrew, MBChB, MSc[a], Roshan Morbia, MD[b], H. Peter Lorenz, MD[a,b],*

KEYWORDS

• Pediatric • Child • Fracture • Facial • Bone • Injury • Surgery

KEY POINTS

• The incidence of head trauma is higher in the pediatric population; however, facial fractures are less prevalent than in the adult population.
• Anatomic and behavioral factors contribute to the increasing incidence of facial fracture with age.
• The decision between operative and nonoperative management is the compromise between pediatric facial growth, and precise reduction and rigid fixation.
• When maxillomandibular fixation is needed, a technique should be adopted that does not damage developing dental tooth buds, such as circummaxillomandibular wiring.

INTRODUCTION

Trauma is the predominant cause of morbidity within the pediatric population. Pediatric trauma results in 12,000 deaths annually in the United States.[1] The incidence of facial trauma in the pediatric population is higher than in the adult population. However, the incidence of facial fracture is lower as a result of reduced mineralization of the facial skeleton, large fat pads, decreased pneumatization of sinuses, and compliant sutures. These anatomic factors allow the facial skeleton to absorb energy without fracturing, and when fracture does occur, it is more likely incomplete, resulting in greenstick injury.

In addition to the unique anatomy of the pediatric patient, future growth and development must be accounted for when addressing injuries. A nonoperative approach is advised whenever possible, and long-term follow-up is mandatory to ensure adequate aesthetic and functional outcomes. The objective of this article is to provide the reader with an understanding of the unique elements of facial fracture management in the pediatric population.

EPIDEMIOLOGY

Facial fractures carry a significant morbidity despite only accounting for 4.6% of pediatric trauma.[2] Considerable force is required to cause a fracture in the pediatric facial skeleton; thus, 55.6% of pediatric facial fracture cases have severe concomitant injuries.[3] Pediatric patients with facial fractures spend twice as long in the hospital and 3 times as long in the intensive care unit (ICU) compared with those without facial fracture.[2]

The most common mechanisms of pediatric facial fracture are road traffic incidents (55.1%), assaults (14.5%), and falls (8.6%).[2] The cause of facial fracture in children correlates with age. Falls are most common among infants and toddlers; road traffic accidents are usually seen in school children, and interpersonal violence (IPV) is most often seen in older teenagers. Age also correlates with the incidence of pediatric facial fracture (**Table 1**).[3] The frequency and severity of injury increase with age, and the prevalence is greater in boys (2–3:1). The incidence of pediatric facial fracture is lowest in 5 year olds (5.6%), and the highest

Disclosure Statement: Drs Andrew and Lorenz have received funding from Hagey Laboratory for Pediatric Regenerative Medicine.

[a] Hagey Laboratory for Pediatric Regenerative Medicine, Division of Plastic Surgery, Department of Surgery, School of Medicine, Stanford University, 257 Campus Drive, Stanford, CA 94305, USA; [b] Division of Plastic Surgery, Department of Surgery, School of Medicine, Stanford University, 770 Welch Road, Suite 400, Stanford, CA 94305, USA

* Corresponding author. Hagey Laboratory for Pediatric Regenerative Medicine, 257 Campus Drive, Stanford, CA 94305.

E-mail address: plorenz@stanford.edu

Table 1
Correlation of age with incidence of pediatric facial fracture

Age Group	0–5 y old	6–11 y old	12–18 y old
Most common mechanism	Falls (43.6%)	Motor vehicle crash (24.9%)	IPV (25.3%)
Operative intervention	28.2%	36.0%	39.4%
ICU admission	28.8%	20.6%	12.9%

Data from Grunwaldt L, Smith DM, Zuckerbraun NS, et al. Pediatric facial fractures: demographics, injury patterns, and associated injuries in 772 consecutive patients. Plast Reconstr Surg 2011;128(6):1263–71.

among teenagers, with 55.9% occurring between 15 and 17 years old.[2,4]

Nonaccidental injuries, although rare, are important to consider in every pediatric facial trauma assessment. Nonaccidental injuries result in head or neck injuries in 50% of cases.[5] Facial fractures caused by IPV are more likely to occur in older, male, non-white, and lower socioeconomic patients.[6] IPV often results in nasal and mandible angle fracture, whereas non–interpersonal violence–related injuries more likely result in skull and orbital fracture. Craniofacial injuries occur in 20% of all pediatric sport-related injuries in the United States.[7] Road traffic accidents are the most common cause of pediatric facial fracture among children, accounting for 50% of cases. Unrestrained children are significantly more likely to sustain facial injury. However, the incidence of facial fracture has significantly reduced since the introduction of seatbelt legislation.[8]

Anatomic site of facial fracture varies according to age in the pediatric population. Nasal fractures are often underreported, most of which do not undergo surgical management.[9] Anatomic distribution of mandible fractures varies with age: condylar head and subcondylar fractures are most common (48%); however, the incidence of condylar fracture decreases with age, whereas body and angle fracture incidence increases.[10,11] Surgical treatment rates for pediatric facial fracture vary greatly, from 25% to 78%.[3] However, older children more often require surgery than younger children.[12]

PREOPERATIVE ASSESSMENT

When managing a child with facial trauma, the Advanced Trauma Life Support protocol should be strictly followed. The assessment consists of the primary survey, resuscitation, secondary survey, diagnostic evaluation, and definitive management.[13] The airway is precarious in children and should be secured at all times. Despite the severity of facial trauma, the child should always be assessed in the structured airway, breathing, circulation, survey approach.

The pediatric population presents exceptional considerations for initial management. Their relative size and surface area to volume ratio puts children at risk for multisystem injury, with potential rapid decompensation due to hypovolemia and hypothermia. A small shoulder roll should be placed to compensate for the occipital prominence in infants and toddlers. Children are at higher risk of spinal cord injury without radiological findings due to their relatively large head and a greater cartilaginous component of the vertebral column, so additional care should be taken in supporting the cervical spine even after radiological clearance.

Nonaccidental injury (NAI) should be suspected if inconsistencies in the history of presentation, prolonged duration between injury and care, noncompliance, or multiple presentations are present. NAI is associated with higher injury severity scores, higher ICU readmission rates, and increased mortality.[14] The head and neck region accounts for more than two-thirds of injuries from abuse.[5] Communication of concerns for NAI to the child protection team is essential.

The head and neck examination should be methodical, fastidious, and consistent. In some instances, the age of the patient limits compliance, and sedation or general anesthesia may be necessary to complete a comprehensive assessment. Examination of all abrasions, lacerations, and contusions should be performed, removing any obstructions, including bandages and secretions. Lacerations should be explored for tissue loss, viability, and depth, while evaluating the reconstructive options and the possibility of using these wounds as surgical access for fracture repair. As much as feasible, facial motor and sensory nerve function should be documented before surgical wound or fracture treatment intervention.

Inspection of the craniofacial skeleton should involve the identification of particular signs that are characteristic for associated facial fractures, such as hypertelorism, Battle sign, malocclusion, trismus, entrapment, raccoon eyes, facial numbness, and otorrhea and/or rhinorrhea. These signs suggest an underlying craniofacial fracture and necessitate radiographic imaging. Palpation of the cranium and facial skeleton should be performed in a methodical superior to inferior fashion, with emphasis on frontal bones, zygomatic arches, orbital rims, oral cavity, and mandibular stability. Otoscopy, rhinoscopy, and ophthalmoscopy are essential to exclude subtle facial injuries. Eye examination can be challenging in the pediatric trauma population. Pupillary reactivity, ocular mobility, globe position, and vision should be assessed. Formal assessment by the ophthalmology team is recommended for all periorbital fractures and any situation with suspected visual loss.

Digital photography plays a vital role in documentation and can assist in counseling families regarding aesthetic challenges as well a supporting multidisciplinary surgical planning. Radiological images should be limited in the pediatric population, and low-dose scanning protocols should be followed.[15] The ability to visualize facial fractures may be limited by anatomic and behavioral limitations. Bony deformity may be obscured by tooth buds, lack of ossification, the predisposition for greenstick-type fractures, and extensive soft tissue injury. Computed tomography (CT) has become the mainstay of diagnostic evaluation for pediatric facial fracture.[12] CT allows for detailed assessment and identification of suspected injuries. CT scans also provide a format for surgical planning and 3-dimensional reconstructions.

UNIQUE FEATURES OF PEDIATRIC FACIAL FRACTURE

In deciding between operative and nonoperative management of pediatric facial fractures, the craniofacial surgeon must weigh the risk of growth disturbance with the benefit of precise reduction and stable fixation. In the immature craniofacial skeleton with minimal displacement, a conservative approach is often preferable. In contrast, a child close to skeletal maturity with significant bone displacement should be managed with open reduction and internal fixation. In accordance with the "functional matrix" principle of Moss and Salentijn,[16] periosteal stripping should be minimalized when fixating the fracture, because the periosteum serves as the main contributor to new bone formation. Hence, extensive periosteal stripping is more likely to result in adverse skeletal development.

To avoid growth disturbance, resorbable plating systems have been proposed in skeletally immature patients. Resorbable plating provides temporary stabilization of bony fracture without the need for a second surgery for plate removal. The blunt tips of the screws and future resorption offer decreased risk to developing teeth and nerve

structures or facial growth. Foreign-body reaction is rare with the resorbable polymers used for facial fracture management.[17] Some surgeons have proposed delayed operative intervention of facial fractures until edema settles. However, because of the enhanced healing of the pediatric skeleton, malunion may be initialized within 3 to 4 days of injury. If the decision is made to operate, the procedure should be performed as soon as localized edema is no longer prohibitive.

SKULL AND FOREHEAD FRACTURES

There is an increased risk of pediatric skull and forehead trauma due to a high cranium to face ratio. Given the lack of protection from pneumatizd frontal sinus in younger children, the incidence of intracranial injury with frontal bone fracture has been reported to be as high as 35% to 64%.[18,19] Cerebrospinal fluid (CSF) leak is also common, occurring in 18% to 36% of frontal bone fractures.[20]

When suspecting a frontal bone fracture, the patient must be evaluated for fracture displacement, CSF leak, intracranial hematoma, deformed facial contour, and frontal-lobe contusion. All dressings should be removed to allow full visualization, and lacerations should be washed to examine. The skull should be thoroughly palpated for any bony or soft tissue defect. Brow examination should include palpation of bony step-offs and paresthesia, and brow or lid ptosis should be documented.

Before pneumatization of the frontal sinus, fractures of the frontal bone or supraorbital ridges are considered to be anterior cranial base fractures.

Operative Approach

The goals of skull and forehead fracture repair include protection of the neurocapsule, dural reconstruction, control of CSF leaks, prevention of posttraumatic infection, and aesthetic restoration of craniofacial contours.

Most pediatric frontal fractures that are minimally or non-displaced can be treated conservatively with adequate follow-up. When frontal fractures are significantly displaced, a surgical approach via a coronal incision in combination with a frontal craniotomy is needed. A combined plastic and neurosurgical approach is often necessary for these complicated procedures. After exposing the fracture, the dura must be inspected. Epidural hematomas are evacuated, and dural lacerations are repaired. When a CSF leak is present with minimal bone displacement, it can be observed and managed with 4 to 7 days of bed rest, possibly with a lumbar drain. Cranialization

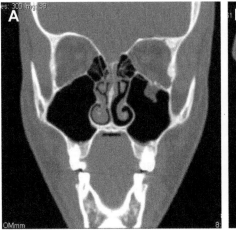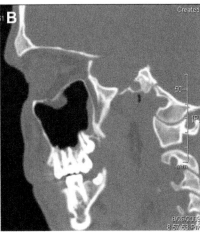

Fig. 1. (*A*) Coronal and (*B*) sagittal CT images demonstrating left orbital floor "trapdoor" fracture with entrapment of orbital soft tissue contents in a 14-year-old male patient.

is performed if the leak persists. In younger children, only resorbable plating systems should be used because metallic hardware can transmigrate endocranially due to calvarial bone growth.

When the frontal sinus is present, the goal of surgical repair is to achieve adequate drainage throughout growth and development. If the posterior wall or inferior drainage system has been severely damaged, then the frontal sinus should be cranialized. To ensure complete separation of the nose from the intracranial cavity, the floor of the sinus should be lined by vascularized tissue, such as a pericranial flap or galeal-frontalis flap. Preservation of the frontal sinus requires long-term follow-up with serial CT scans to ensure adequate drainage. Nasofrontal duct stents can be placed if there are concerns with drainage. Endoscopic sinus surgery can be done to open duct/drainage.

ORBITAL FRACTURE

Orbital fractures occur as a result of 2 mechanisms. First, the "hydraulic" theory suggests that direct pressure and compression force of the globe directly fracture the thin bone of the orbital wall, in particular, the inferior and medial walls resulting in orbital blowout.[21] Second, the "bone conduction" theory describes the distribution of energy absorbed at the orbital rim resulting in buckling of the floor with fracture at the weakest point.[22]

Pediatric orbital fractures are clinically distinct from adult orbital fractures. Fractures of the supraorbital rim are often classified as skull base fractures because they include the frontal bones before sinus pneumatization. The incidence of orbital roof fractures is highest before the age of

7 years, after which age a decrease in the neurocranium to viscerocranium ratio occurs, and the development of the frontal sinus "crumple zone" begins. The relatively large neurocranium in young children increases the susceptibility of neurologic injury due to orbital fracture. In contrast, older patients are more likely to sustain midface and ophthalmic injury. Routine ophthalmologic consultation should be obtained in any patient with periorbital trauma. Inspection for subconjunctival hemorrhage and extraocular muscle movement range, including diplopia, should be performed. Superior orbital fissure syndrome, which comprises internal and external ophthalmoplegia, proptosis, and CN VI paresthesia, should be treated as an emergency. If superior orbital fissure syndrome occurs in combination with blindness, it is described as orbital apex syndrome.

The orbital floor "trapdoor" fracture occurs most commonly in children. "Trapdoor" fracture occurs when the transient opening in the orbital floor entraps the orbital contents, including the inferior rectus muscle (**Fig. 1**). The signs of entrapment include nausea, vomiting, and oculocardiac reflex. Inferior orbital entrapment is a clinical diagnosis and cannot be excluded by imaging studies alone. Forced duction testing is a useful way of distinguishing diplopia of entrapment from pseudoentrapment from nerve injury due to localized swelling. Forced duction testing in children is often performed under general anesthesia. The conjunctiva is grasped with forceps close to the limbus and is moved away from the side of suspected entrapment. Medial wall fractures carry a significant but reduced risk of entrapment involving the medial rectus muscle. Caution should be taken when considering a possible white-eyed blowout

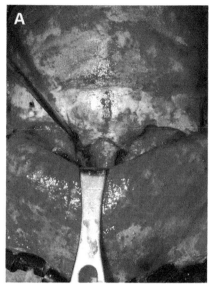
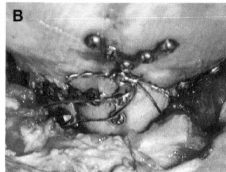

Fig. 2. Bicoronal approach to a bilateral displaced NOE fracture in a 13-year-old patient. (*A*) Displaced NOE fractures. (*B*). Reduced and plated NOE fractures and transnasal medial canthoplasty wires.

fracture. In these patients, the eye appears uninjured without subconjunctival hemorrhage; however, the child will have severe restriction of gaze secondary to soft tissue entrapment in the trapdoor fracture. The soft tissue herniation may not be readily visible on CT. The bony fracture line is usually difficult to image on CT. Entrapment in the white-eyed blowout fracture is often associated with the oculocardiac reflex (bradycardia, nausea, and syncope), which is an absolute indication for urgent surgical intervention.

Operative Technique

In the absence of entrapment or acute globe malposition, management is often conservative. The goals of orbital fracture treatment include the restoration of globe position with correction of diplopia and release of entrapment. If open reduction internal fixation (ORIF) is necessary, some investigators have suggested that the transconjunctival approach is preferred for good cosmesis and a lower risk of ectropion.[23] If lateral exposure is necessary, a subciliary or midlid incision with lateral "crow's foot" extension avoids the lateral cantholysis that may be necessary with a transconjunctival incision and affords generous exposure extending to the lateral-superior orbital rim/orbit. If medial exposure is necessary, a transcaruncular approach is performed, often obviating a coronal incision. A gingival buccal sulcus incision can be added if necessary. Herniated tissues are reduced from the sinus; the fracture is cleared of debris, and stable edges for fixation and grafting are identified. After adequate exposure and relocation of

herniated soft tissue, the stable bony ledges of the fracture are spanned with plates or bone grafts; many craniofacial surgeons use autologous material, such as split calvarial bone fragments, iliac crest, or rib grafts, for orbital reconstruction of the growing facial skeleton. Absorbable plates and mesh are used for fixation as needed.

Possible complications include retrobulbar hematoma, orbital cellulitis, lid malposition, enophthalmos, and persistent diplopia. Retrobulbar hematoma is sight threatening and presents with pain, proptosis, and internal ophthalmoplegia and should be managed with urgent lateral cantholysis for orbital decompression.

NASAL AND NASOETHMOIDAL FRACTURE

Nasal fractures are common among children. The presence of soft cartilage and incompletely ossified nasal bone means that pediatric nasal fractures are often missed. The younger child has a reduced risk of nasal bone fracture due to decreased rostral projection, shorter dorsum, larger cartilaginous portion, and increased bony compliance. The incidence peaks in adolescence because of anatomy and behavioral factors.[4]

Naso-orbital ethmoidal (NOE) fractures are rare in the pediatric population and occur as a result of high-energy trauma. Unlike in adults, patterns of fracture are different due to proportional difference in midface to neurocranium and the lack of pneumatization of the frontal sinus. Pediatric NOE fractures are characterized by posterior and lateral displacement of nasal bones and medial orbital wall, including the ethmoid (**Fig. 2**). The medial canthus inserts at the medial orbital wall, resulting in potential traumatic telecanthus; this may not be apparent until 7 to 10 days after injury when edema has subsided.

Physical examination must include endonasal examination to rule out septal hematoma. Septal hematoma requires immediate intervention with mucoperiosteal incision. Caution should be taken to avoid overlapping bilateral incisions resulting in potential septal perforation. Suture quilting and postoperative intranasal splints should be used to compress the mucoperichondrium to obliterate any dead space. Non-displaced nasal fracture may be managed with external splint. The septum is an important center for midface growth. Because of the potential risks of restricted facial growth, definitive open management of displaced nasal fractures is often delayed until skeletal maturity. However, displaced nasal bone fractures still require closed reduction, which is best performed under general anesthesia. Ash forceps are used to relocate the septum, and a Goldman elevator is used to reduce nasal bones, as is done in adults. Because of the rapid healing ability of children, closed reduction should be performed 3 to 7 days after injury. Pediatric open septorhinoplasty is typically reserved for severely displaced fractures, sleep apnea, and chronic refractory sinus disease.

Pediatric NOE fractures with telecanthus should have the intercanthal distance restored to age-specific standards; this is often performed by reduction of the medial orbital rims. Medial canthal tendons are reattached with transnasal wires passing superiorly and posteriorly to the posterior lacrimal crest. As in nasal fractures, the likelihood of additional secondary surgery in adolescence is high due to factors related to facial skeletal growth.

Nasal fracture may result in several deformities. Nasal fractures in children may affect facial skeleton growth, resulting in nasal hypoplasia. Nasal deviation may occur as a result of cartilaginous warping or incomplete reduction. If untreated, a septal hematoma may result in septal thickening or perforation, ultimately developing into a saddle-nose deformity.

MIDFACE/ZYGOMATICOMAXILLARY FRACTURES

Classical Le Fort midface fractures are rare in children due to an undeveloped buttress system, small paranasal sinuses, and unerupted tooth buds. Examination may reveal a mobile midface, palpable bony step-offs, and malocclusion. Zygomaticomaxillary complex (ZMC) fractures often present with malar flattening, enophthalmos, and lateral canthal dystopia (**Fig. 3**). CT is the gold-standard imaging modality for midface fracture confirmation because soft tissue swelling can often obscure midface deformity.

The treatment goals of surgery in pediatric midface fractures are to achieve accurate reduction and sufficiently stable fixation to permit bone healing while avoiding disturbance to future growth. Minimally displaced and greenstick midface fractures are often managed nonoperatively, especially in younger children. Displaced or unstable maxillary fractures require either closed reduction with mandibulomaxillary fixation or ORIF. Rigidity and length of fixation are less than in adults. When performing ORIF, care must be taken to avoid injury to the developing tooth buds when plating fractures.

The operative goals in ZMC fracture surgery are correction of malocclusion and restoration of malar prominence. Access to the zygomaticofrontal (ZF) suture may be achieved through a brow incision or upper lid blepharoplasty incision. Generally, 3-point fixation is required at the ZF suture, inferior orbital rim, and zygomaticomaxillary buttress. Maxillary fractures may result in nasolacrimal obstruction or malocclusion. Pediatric patients with maxillomandibular fixation (MMF) are at risk of malnutrition.

MANDIBLE

Children with mandible fractures are at risk of airway compromise. The airway must be secured during initial management; at times, endotracheal intubation or a surgical airway may be necessary to achieve this. CT imaging of the head and neck are also necessary to exclude concomitant injuries. Furthermore, the panorex has largely been superseded by CT imaging on the mandible.

Intraoral lacerations, ecchymosis, and edema may suggest an underlying mandibular fracture. Paresthesia of the inferior alveolar nerve can occur in displaced fractures. A thorough intraoral examination must be performed, and subjective malocclusion may be noted. Drooling and trismus may also be noted. Bimanual examination of the mandible may demonstrate bony step-offs. The external auditory canal may show bleeding and ecchymosis. Palpation of the TMJ at the external auditory canal during jaw movement may demonstrate crepitation or a displaced condylar head. Trismus causing malocclusion with no or minimal bony displacement can be seen in children. CT imaging is critical to determine if significant displacement is present.

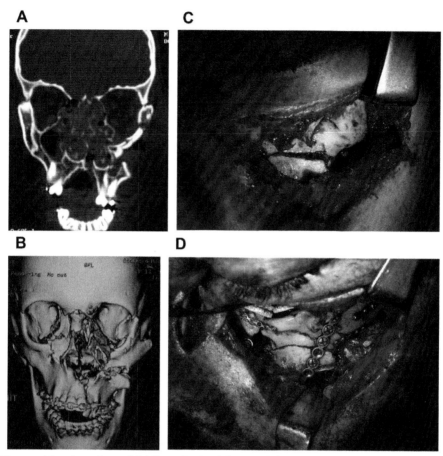

Fig. 3. A 13-year-old male patient with bilateral NOE, left ZMC, left orbital floor, palate, and left Le Fort I fractures. (*A*) Coronal CT and (*B*) 3-dimensional reconstruction images. (*C*) Left zygomatic body with orbital floor blowout fracture intraoperatively. Existing laceration used for fracture exposure. (*D*) Fixation of zygomatic bone and split calvarial bone grafts to orbital floor.

The treatment goals are to achieve restoration of normal occlusion and to achieve bony union without interrupting potential facial growth development. In the developing jaw, future orthodontic correction allows for minor occlusal discrepancies rather than aggressive corrective operative treatment. If possible, the patient's dentist and orthodontist should be contacted to obtain any preinjury dental records.

A minimally displaced mandibular fracture may be managed with jaw rest and immobilization with a jaw compression wrap or cervical collar as well as a liquid diet. Dentoalveolar fractures can often be managed with occlusive splinting, arch bars, and/or bonded wires. Minor malocclusion should be managed orthodontically after bony healing is finished. Applying MMF in children during primary and mixed dentition phases may be challenging but can be safely practiced.[24] When MMF is needed during these phases, a technique should be adopted that does not damage

developing dental tooth buds such as circummaxillomandibular wiring. In addition, the primary dentition does not hold interproximal space wires for arch bars well. During mixed dentition, MMF plating systems are not advised due to developing tooth buds (**Fig. 4**). Correlation with CT images and displacement is mandatory. Fractures can be managed with a liquid diet and frequent examination, with surgery reserved for situations in which occlusion is not improving.

Mandibular condyles are growth centers that are sensitive to disruptions in blood supply and prone to ankyloses with fracture trauma and/or surgery.[25] Intracapsular fractures, high condylar neck fractures, and coronoid fractures should be managed conservatively to minimize these complications. Early range-of-motion exercises should be started at 3 to 5 days after injury with physiotherapy. Unilateral condylar neck fractures and bilateral condylar neck fractures are often managed conservatively with a liquid diet.

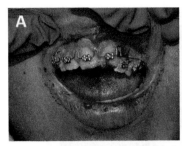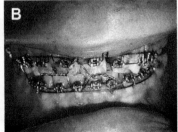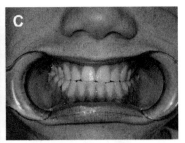

Fig. 4. Preexisting orthodontic appliances can be used to establish MMF. (A) Preoperative photograph. (B) Postoperative photograph with patient in wire loop MMF. (C) Long-term outcome.

However, in older patients, ORIF of one side is reasonable to avoid potential temporomandibular joint (TMJ) dysfunction and also to restore occlusion. Open management is also recommended when a foreign body is in the TMJ or when condylar displacement into the middle cranial fossa occurs. ORIF should be performed through preexisting lacerations with or without intraoral approach to fully expose the fracture sites and place rigid fixation. For body and angle fractures, the standard anterior sulcus incision should be performed, leaving a cuff of mentalis muscle attached to the upper edge of the incision to avoid a witch's chin deformity. Care should be taken to dissect out the mental nerve.

The pediatric mandible is able to remodel under masticatory forces, and the potential for orthodontic correction is also present. The remodeling capability of the pediatric mandible allows for imperfect reduction and occlusion often to be acceptable in order to preserve tooth follicle development. If internal bony fixation is necessary in younger patients, then monocortical screws should be used and hardware should be placed on the inferior mandibular border to avoid the developing tooth buds.

SUMMARY

The structure and topography of the pediatric craniofacial skeleton are profoundly different from the mature skull. Consequently, the pediatric facial skeleton responds differently to traumatic force. Although the incidence of pediatric facial trauma is higher than in the adult population, the incidence of facial fracture is significantly lower. The management options for pediatric craniofacial fracture can be controversial; thus, evaluation and operative approaches are uniquely based on the patient's age and development. Fracture management in younger patients is often more conservative due to potential growth impairment and greater remodeling. As the facial skeleton matures, more conventional surgical approaches

become appropriate. Long-term growth patterns of children after facial fracture remain unpredictable, emphasizing the need for long-term follow-up and further multicenter, controlled trials.

REFERENCES

1. Borse N, Sleet DA. CDC childhood injury report patterns of unintentional injuries among 0-to 19-year olds in the United States, 2000-2006. Fam Community Health 2009;32(2):189.
2. Imahara SD, Hopper RA, Wang J, et al. Patterns and outcomes of pediatric facial fractures in the United States: a survey of the national trauma data bank. J Am Coll Surg 2008;207(5):710–6.
3. Grunwaldt L, Smith DM, Zuckerbraun NS, et al. Pediatric facial fractures: demographics, injury patterns, and associated injuries in 772 consecutive patients. Plast Reconstr Surg 2011;128(6):1263–71.
4. Vyas RM, Dickinson BP, Wasson KL, et al. Pediatric facial fractures: current national incidence, distribution, and health care resource use. J Craniofac Surg 2008;19(2):339–49.
5. Ryan ML, Thorson CM, Otero CA, et al. Pediatric facial trauma: a review of guidelines for assessment, evaluation, and management in the emergency department. J Craniofac Surg 2011;22(4):1183–9.
6. Mericli AF, DeCesare GE, Zuckerbraun NS, et al. Pediatric craniofacial fractures due to violence: comparing violent and nonviolent mechanisms of injury. J Craniofac Surg 2011;22(4):1342–7.
7. Afrooz PN, Grunwaldt LJ, Zanoun RR, et al. Pediatric facial fractures: occurrence of concussion and relation to fracture patterns. J Craniofac Surg 2012; 23(5):1270–3.
8. Cox D, Vincent DG, McGwin G, et al. Effect of restraint systems on maxillofacial injury in frontal motor vehicle collisions. J Oral Maxillofac Surg 2004;62(5): 571–5.
9. Kim SH, Lee SH, Cho PD. Analysis of 809 facial bone fractures in a pediatric and adolescent population. Arch Plast Surg 2012;39(6):606–11.
10. Smith DM, Bykowski MR, Cray JJ, et al. 215 mandible fractures in 120 children: demographics,

treatment, outcomes, and early growth data. Plast Reconstr Surg 2013;131(6):1348–58.

11. Smartt JM, Low DW, Bartlett SP. The pediatric mandible: II. management of traumatic injury or fracture. Plast Reconstr Surg 2005;116(2):28e–41e.

12. Zimmermann CE, Troulis MJ, Kaban LB. Pediatric facial fractures: recent advances in prevention, diagnosis and management (vol 35, pg 2, 2006). Int J Oral Maxillofac Surg 2006;35(1):1–13.

13. Hoppe IC, Kordahi AM, Paik AM, et al. Examination of life-threatening injuries in 431 pediatric facial fractures at a level 1 trauma center. J Craniofac Surg 2014;25(5):1825–8.

14. Davidson EH, Schuster L, Rottgers SA, et al. Severe pediatric midface trauma: a prospective study of growth and development. J Craniofac Surg 2015; 26(5):1523–8.

15. Tsiklakis K, Donta C, Gavala S, et al. Dose reduction in maxillofacial imaging using low dose Cone Beam CT. Eur J Radiol 2005;56(3):413–7.

16. Moss ML, Salentijn L. The primary role of functional matrices in facial growth. Am J Orthod 1969;55(6): 566–77.

17. Eppley BL. Use of resorbable plates and screws in pediatric facial fractures. J Oral Maxillofac Surg 2005;63(3):385–91.

18. Whatley WS, Allison DW, Chandra RK, et al. Frontal sinus fractures in children. Laryngoscope 2005; 115(10):1741–5.

19. Gerbino G, Roccia F, Benech A, et al. Analysis of 158 frontal sinus fractures: current surgical management and complications. J Craniomaxillofac Surg 2000;28(3):133–9.

20. Jones DT, Mcgill TJ, Healy GB. Cerebrospinal fistulas in children. Laryngoscope 1992;102(4):443–6.

21. Erling BF, Iliff N, Robertson B, et al. Footprints of the globe: a practical look at the mechanism of orbital blowout fractures, with a revisit to the work of Raymond Pfeiffer. Plast Reconstr Surg 1999;103(4): 1313–6.

22. Anderson RL, Panje WR, Gross CE. Optic-nerve blindness following blunt forehead trauma. Ophthalmology 1982;89(5):445–55.

23. Lorenz HP, Longaker MT, Kawamoto HK Jr. Primary and secondary orbit surgery: the transconjunctival approach. Plast Reconstr Surg 1999;103(4):1124–8.

24. Naran S, Keating J, Natali M, et al. The safe and efficacious use of arch bars in patients during primary and mixed dentition: a challenge to conventional teaching. Plast Reconstr Surg 2014;133(2):364–6.

25. Blackwood HJ. Vascularization of condylar cartilage of human mandible. J Anat 1965;99:551–63.

Pierre Robin Sequence

Sun T. Hsieh, MS, MD[a], Albert S. Woo, MD[b],*

KEYWORDS

- Pierre Robin sequence • Cleft palate • Micrognathia • Glossoptosis • Distraction

KEY POINTS

- Pierre Robin sequence (PRS) consists of the clinical triad of micrognathia, glossoptosis, and airway compromise with variable inclusion of cleft palate.
- Management of airway obstruction in PRS consists of nonsurgical maneuvers, such as prone positioning and nasopharyngeal stenting; surgical management includes mandibular distraction and tongue-lip adhesion.
- Diagnostic evaluation of patients with PRS includes nasoendoscopy and bronchoscopy for the airway and a multidisciplinary approach for multisystemic anomalies in syndromic patients.

 Video content accompanies this article at http://www.plasticsurgery.theclinics.com.

INTRODUCTION

Pierre Robin sequence (PRS) consists of the clinical triad of congenital micrognathia, glossoptosis, and airway obstruction with variable inclusion of a cleft palate (**Fig. 1**). When this constellation of findings occurs in the absence of other congenital anomalies, it is termed isolated PRS; however, PRS oftentimes finds itself a component of a more complex syndromic picture. This phenotypic heterogeneity arises from a permutation of mechanical, genetic, and environmental derangements. The variable complexity of the patient presentation lends itself to a multidisciplinary approach in uncovering the diagnosis, managing the airway obstruction, optimizing the feeding, and addressing the multisystemic abnormalities intrinsic to the syndromic patient. Although nearly a century has passed since the description of Robin's eponymous triad, incongruities remain regarding treatment protocols among different centers. This lack of consensus reflects the high degree of difficulty in the management of such a diverse patient population, a challenge that cannot be overstated.

HISTORICAL PERSPECTIVE

In 1835, Von Siebold described a case of micrognathia, microglossia, and glossoptosis in an infant who ultimately succumbed to asphyxia.[1] Nearly a century later, French stomatologist Pierre Robin's[2] seminal 1923 paper described the same constellation of findings, namely glossoptosis in the presence of micrognathia, highlighting the dire consequences to the airway. The historical literature is littered with various authors who separately encountered and described this set of findings, including St. Hillaire in 1822, Fäsebeck in 1842, Fairbairn in 1846, and Shukowski in 1911.[3] Ultimately, these collections of findings assumed the eponymous title of Pierre Robin sequence.

EPIDEMIOLOGY

The incidence of PRS ranges from 1 in 8000 to 1 in 14,000.[4,5] Mortality for infants with PRS ranges from 1.7% to 11.3%; the rate increases to 26% when examining only the subset of syndromic patients.[6] Although cleft palate is not a strict criterion

---

Disclosure Statement: The authors have nothing to disclose.
[a] Department of Plastic Surgery, Rhode Island Hospital, The Warren Alpert Medical School of Brown University, 2 Dudley Street, Suite 500, Providence, RI 02905, USA; [b] Pediatric Plastic Surgery, Craniofacial Program, Rhode Island Hospital, The Warren Alpert Medical School of Brown University, 2 Dudley Street, Suite 180, Providence, RI 02905, USA
* Corresponding author.
E-mail address: albertswoo@gmail.com

Clin Plastic Surg 46 (2019) 249–259
https://doi.org/10.1016/j.cps.2018.11.010

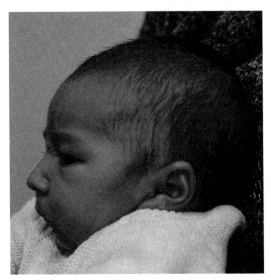

Fig. 1. Lateral view of infant with PRS, which consists of the clinical triad of retromicrognathia, glossoptosis, and airway compromise with variable inclusion of a cleft palate.

for the diagnosis of PRS, 85% of these patients present with a concomitant cleft.[4] The incidence of these patients presenting with an associated syndrome is 38% to 44%. Male and female individuals are affected at an equal rate.[4,5,7]

INTRAUTERINE DEVELOPMENT

Craniofacial morphogenesis begins with delamination of neural crest cells from the dorsal neural tube into ventral pharyngeal arches.[8,9] The first pharyngeal arch forms the maxilla and mandible through intramembranous ossification. The Meckel cartilage serves as the initial scaffold onto which mandibular intramembranous ossification occurs, orienting mandibular growth in a proximo-distal configuration.

Maxillary development occurs concomitantly with mandibular outgrowth. Lateral palatal shelves extend from the maxillary arches at approximately the seventh week of gestation and begin to grow in a sagittal plane adjacent to the tongue.[8]

As mandibular outgrowth continues, the tongue is flattened and distracted anteriorly by the genioglossus, originating on the lingual surface of the mandible.[8] This facilitates reorientation of sagittal palatal shelves into a transverse plane. The medial edge epithelia fuse in coordinated fashion in an anterior-to-posterior direction on the eighth week, as illustrated in **Fig. 2**.

Classically, the inciting insult in PRS is a micrognathic mandible that obligates retropositioning of the tongue base, predisposing the infant to glottic airway compromise. Inability of the tongue base to

descend from the roof of the nasopharynx causes a physical blockade to palate formation, preventing appropriate elevation, medialization, and fusion of the palatal shelves.[8]

GENETIC FINDINGS

There is no classic causal relationship between PRS and a single genetic mutation, but rather a wide swath of genetic errors that have been associated with a variety of phenotypic presentations. **Box 1** contains a list of associated syndromes.

Approximately 26% to 83% of PRS diagnoses are part of a syndrome, most commonly Stickler syndrome, 22q11.2 Deletion Syndrome, Treacher Collins syndrome, and Campomelic Dysplasia, among others.[10,11] Approximately 11% to 18% of patients with PRS are diagnosed with Stickler syndrome, a connective tissue disorder impacting collagen metabolism.[8] Ocular findings are most prominent, presenting as myopia, vitreous abnormalities, glaucoma, retinal detachment, and cataracts. Skeletal sequelae, hearing loss, and craniofacial anomalies may be present. Velocardiofacial syndrome accounts for approximately 11% of patients with PRS.[10] Now known as 22q11.2 Deletion Syndrome, findings include learning disability, micrognathia, cleft palate, long philtrum, conductive hearing loss, hypoparathyroidism, and thymic aplasia.

DIAGNOSIS AND INITIAL MANAGEMENT

Patients with PRS frequently have other systemic anomalies that warrant a multidisciplinary approach to their diagnosis and management.[12] A comprehensive evaluation may require involvement of specialties such as maternal-fetal medicine, genetics, neonatology, pulmonary and sleep medicine, developmental pediatrics, plastic surgery, oral surgery, orthodontics, dentistry, otolaryngology, ophthalmology, pediatric surgery, cardiology, speech pathology, feeding specialists, audiology, and neurology.

PRENATAL IMAGING

Diagnostic workup may start in the prenatal period with ultrasound or MRI.[12] Micrognathia may be difficult to diagnose via ultrasound, with sensitivity of 72.7%.[13] Normalization of the mandibular anteroposterior length by the biparietal skull width creates a jaw index, which improves ultrasound sensitivity to 100% and specificity to 98.1%.[14] The positive predictive value for diagnosing PRS versus isolated micrognathia correlates directly with the maxillomandibular discrepancy.[13,15] Polyhydramnios is

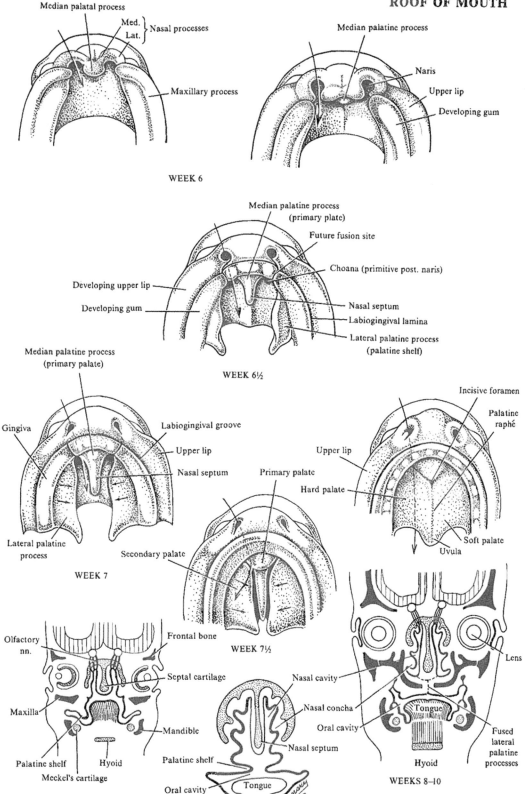

Fig. 2. Normal intrauterine development of primary and secondary palate with reorientation of the palatal shelves from a vertical to horizontal position. A retrognathic mandible leads to retropositioning of the tongue, which impedes this fusion process. (*From* https://discovery.lifemapsc.com/library/review-of-medical-embryology/chapter-55-development-of-the-palate. Accessed May 1, 2018.)

Box 1
List of syndromes most frequently associated with Pierre Robin sequence

Associated Syndromes

Stickler syndrome

22q11.2 Deletion syndrome

Treacher Collins syndrome

Campomelic dysplasia

Marshall syndrome

Nager syndrome

Miller syndrome

Kabuki syndrome

Catel-Manske syndrome

Congenital myotonic dystrophy

Carey-Fineman-Ziter syndrome

Fetal alcohol syndrome

Maternal diabetes

Spondyloepiphyseal dysplasia congenita

Hemifacial microsomia

Glass syndrome

Mandibulofacial dysostosis

---

associated with impaired swallowing secondary to glossoptosis.

AIRWAY EVALUATION

Airway obstruction is life-threatening for the neonate. Prolonged obstruction results in hypoxia, apnea, respiratory tract infections, aspiration, compromised feeding, and failure to thrive.[16] Chronic hypoxia leads to increased pulmonary vascular resistance, cor pulmonale, heart failure, and cerebral hypoxia.[16]

Robin[2] attributed neonatal airway compromise to posterior displacement of the tongue base. This decreases the cross-sectional area of the oropharynx, limiting mass flow rate of oxygen during respiration and predisposing the upper airway to collapse during inspiration.[17]

Physical examination provides a clinical gestalt of the patient's respiratory effort through observations of stridor, positional retraction of the chest and neck, positional desaturation, cyanosis, and feeding difficulty (Video 1).[6] Nasopharyngoscopy may reveal synchronous lesions, such as subglottic stenosis, laryngomalacia, tracheomalacia, bronchomalacia, choanal atresia, tracheal stenosis, and aspiration bronchitis.[18]

Polysomnography quantifies obstruction events and gas exchange disturbances, although utility of the apnea-hypopnea index (AHI) is limited by the lack of standardized neonatal normative values.[13] Sleep studies differentiate between obstructive and central sleep apnea, the latter prompting greater consideration before surgical intervention. Polysomnography as a diagnostic tool is not uniformly adopted. Opponents highlight the absence of an objective threshold with which to gauge the clinical severity of the airway obstruction.[13] Syndromic patients may be longitudinally assessed through serial polysomnography, nasopharyngoscopy, and physical examination as they mature.

FEEDING

Feeding may be dysfunctional secondary to the cleft palate (if present), hypoplastic mandible, and dynamic exacerbation of airway obstruction. Speech pathology monitors feeding sessions for signs of dysphagia, such as coughing, choking, or feeding refusal.[13] Videofluoroscopy, nasoendoscopy, and swallowing studies aid in evaluating dynamic function.

Supplemental feeding is required in 38% to 62% of patients with PRS.[6,13] Temporary nasogastric tube feeding may suffice; however, syndromic patients may develop chronic feeding difficulty, requiring placement of a gastrostomy tube. Tongue-lip adhesion has a nearly threefold risk of eventual gastrostomy tube placement when compared with mandibular distraction.[19] Average weight gain of 20 to 30 g/d is considered satisfactory for the neonate.[20,21] Consistent weight gain allows for transitioning of continuous nasogastric tube feeding to bolus feeds, and eventual oral intake.[19] Oral feeding and swallowing training should be implemented to limit oral aversion. The pediatric gastroenterologist may longitudinally follow the patient to ensure appropriate growth and development.

MANAGEMENT

Treatment of PRS may be divided into nonsurgical and surgical methodologies. Protocols vary across different centers and may be a function of individual surgeons' training and experience, each with their own criteria for pursuing surgical versus nonsurgical intervention.

NONSURGICAL MANAGEMENT

Airway obstruction is initially addressed via prone or lateral positioning with a success rate of 70%.[22] Should the obstruction prove recalcitrant, a nasopharyngeal stent may be placed to mitigate the retroglottic obstruction (**Fig. 3**). Custom stents tailored to the infant's weight may minimize dead

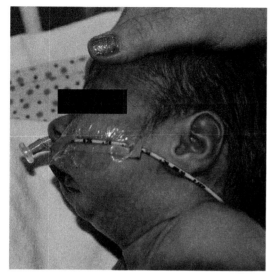

Fig. 3. A nasopharyngeal stent may be used to maintain the retroglottic airway should prone and lateral positioning prove insufficient in relieving retroglottic airway obstruction.

space and permit delivery of supplemental oxygen via nasal cannulas.[23] Positioning and nasopharyngeal stenting alone may be sufficient in infants who maintain a weight above the 25th percentile and have an AHI less than 19.2 events per hour.[24] Supportive stenting may last 2 to 4 months and can continue at home.

Noninvasive continuous positive airway pressure (CPAP) can obviate the need for surgical intervention in a subset of infants with moderate obstruction who can breathe spontaneously while possessing an AHI greater than 10.[25] Once initiated, CPAP is weaned to use only during sleep periods over a period of 1 to 2 weeks, and may be applied for up to 6 months.[25]

Should a noninvasive airway prove inadequate, the patient may undergo endotracheal intubation or placement of a laryngeal mask airway.

SURGICAL MANAGEMENT
Tongue-Lip Adhesion

Tongue-lip adhesion (TLA) acts to increase the cross-sectional area of the oropharyngeal airway by anteriorly tethering the posteriorly displaced tongue base to the hypoplastic mandible. Its indication is limited to when upper and lower airway evaluation has excluded additional subglottic, synchronous lesions. Some view TLA as a first-line surgical treatment for those who fail nonoperative management.

The procedure begins with placement of anterior traction sutures at the lateral aspects of the tongue.[26] The frenulum is released if found to limit

outward movement. The ventral tongue is coapted to the lower lip mucosa and the contact area is identified. A rectangular inferiorly based lower lip musculo-mucosal flap and a congruent superiorly based ventral tongue flap are developed, measuring approximately 2 × 1 cm each (**Fig. 4**). Attention must be paid to avoid injury to the submandibular and sublingual ducts.[27] The leading edge of the lip flap is sutured to the inferior edge of the tongue wound, the exposed labial muscle is sutured to the lingual muscles, and the leading edge of the tongue flap is sutured to the superior edge of the lip wound, in sequential fashion. Apposition of the muscular planes is critical to minimizing risk of dehiscence. Retention sutures secure the tongue base to the lingual surface of the mandible, exiting through the submenton and tied over a button to preserve the underlying skin (**Fig. 5**).[27,28] Endoscopic evaluation of the airway confirms resolution of the retroglottic obstruction. Nasopharyngeal stenting is performed for 2 to 3 days to account for postoperative edema.[28] Nasogastric feeds should be administered for a week to prevent contamination of the wound during the acute healing phase.[28] Muscular adhesion occurs over 2 weeks, after which the retention sutures are released. Division of the TLA occurs between 12 and 18 months postoperatively either concomitantly or in sequence with palate repair.[26] TLA has a success rate of 71% to 89% in relieving the airway obstruction.[26,29]

Complications from TLA include dehiscence, abnormal eruption of deciduous incisors, infection, lip scarring, and tongue edema.[26] The former has largely been mitigated through modifications by Rutledge in the 1960s, with dehiscence rates at 4.2% to 17.2%. Mucosa-only adhesions have reported dehiscence rates of 41.6%.[30] Persistent airway obstruction following TLA on up to 20% of cases likely stems from a failure of elucidating the complete etiology of airway obstruction beyond the tongue base.

AHI can be improved from 30.8 to 15.4 events per hour following TLA.[31] TLA has been shown to improve mean lowest oxygen saturation from 75.8% to 84.4% and mean oxygen saturation from 90.8% to 95%. Feeding outcomes remain disparate with 0% to 54% of infants requiring eventual gastrostomy tube placement depending on the study.[18,26,32]

Floor of Mouth Release

Subperiosteal floor of mouth release (FMR) is based on the assertion that airway obstruction occurs due to a posterior rotation of the tongue secondary to abnormally tight attachments of lingual

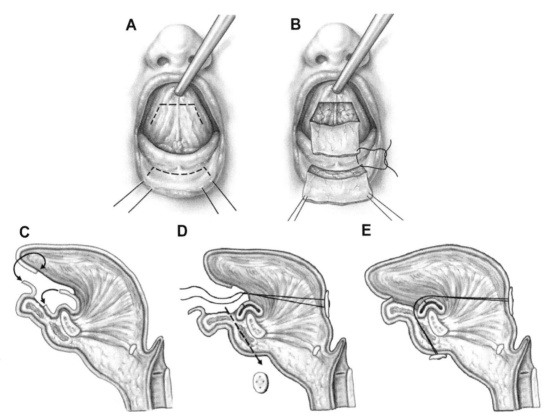

Fig. 4. TLA acts to increase the cross-sectional area of the oropharyngeal airway by anteriorly tethering the posteriorly displaced tongue base to the hypoplastic mandible. A rectangular inferiorly based lower lip musculo-mucosal flap (*A, B*) and a congruent superiorly based ventral tongue flap (*C, D*) are developed and approximated to each other (*E*). (*From* Qaqish C, Caccamese J. The tongue-lip adhesion. Operat Tech Otolaryngol Head Neck Surg 2009;20(4):274–7; with permission.)

musculature onto the lingual mandible.[33] Release of anterior belly of the digastric, myohyoid, genio-hyoid, and genioglossus insertions facilitates de-rotation of the tongue.

Caouette-Laberge and colleagues[34] reported an 84% success rate in infants developing indepen-dence from nasopharyngeal stenting following FMR and a decrease in the AHI from 46.5 to

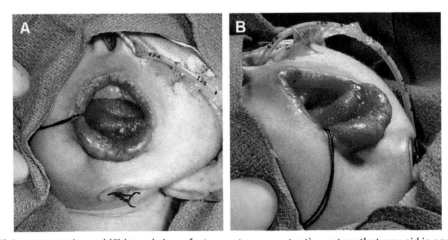

Fig. 5. (*A*) Anteroposterior and (*B*) lateral view of a transcutaneous retention suture that may aid in apposing the tongue base to the lingual surface of the mandible. The button dissipates the chronic stress of the suture and minimizes injury to the skin.

17.4. Gastrostomy feeding was able to be avoided in 73% of cases, with half of patients being orally fed within 11 days postoperatively.

Mandibular Distraction Osteogenesis

McCarthy and colleagues[35] published their experience with mandibular distraction osteogenesis (MDO) on a series of patients with congenital mandibular hypoplasia in 1992, introducing the technique to the field of craniofacial surgery. In the decades since, MDO has experienced wider acceptance among the craniofacial community for treatment of mandibular hypoplasia.[35]

Distraction devices are available in external or semi-buried internal forms. External devices allow for multiple vectors of distraction that can be adjusted following the initial osteotomy and greater distraction length (**Fig. 6**).[36] Disadvantages include buccal scarring, risk of pin dislodgement, decreased precision, greater relapse, patient discomfort, and pin site infections.[36]

Alternatively, distraction can be performed by placement of internal devices. By their nature, internal distractors are less conspicuous with lower scar burden; however, they provide only univector distraction and require precise preoperative planning. Nonresorbable devices require a second surgery for removal. Advantages include patient comfort, prolonged retention period for optimal ossification, and decreased risk of pin site infection.[36]

A brief description of the distractor placement is given. Illustrative photos are shown in **Fig. 7**. A submandibular Risdon incision is made. Dissection continues through the platysma, avoiding injury to the facial vessels and marginal mandibular branch of the facial nerve. The periosteum is incised and a subperiosteal plane is developed, exposing the coronoid and antegonial notch as reference. Distraction vector may be sagittal, vertical oblique, or obtuse depending on the degree of vertical deficiency and occlusal relationship.

A 270° osteotomy is completed of the anterior, posterior, and buccal cortices with a conventional or piezoelectric saw, taking care to spare the inferior alveolar nerve. The internal distraction device is secured with monocortical screws, and the lingual osteotomy is completed. Initial activation of the distractor confirms bony separation and the bony edges are then returned to their original positions. The soft tissue is closed.

Osteotomy design may be aided by virtual surgical planning to minimize injury to developing tooth buds and the inferior alveolar nerve.[37] Configurations include linear oblique, inverted-L, and multiangular. The inverted-L osteotomy is frequently advocated because it proceeds distal to the tooth buds, better preserving these structures.[37] While damage to deciduous teeth can be minimized with imaging and planning, injury to permanent dentition is difficult to predict.

In neonatal MDO, our institution begins the process of distraction the day after surgery at a rate of 2 mm/d. Older patients are allowed a latency period of 2 to 5 days followed by distraction rate of 1 mm/d. The former accelerates the process of distraction, allowing extubation within approximately 1 week postoperatively. The patient is closely monitored during the distraction phase with a goal of moderate prognathism. In the neonate, it is the common practice of Dr Woo AS to attempt 25 to 30 mm of distraction. Once distraction is completed, the externalized portion of the distractor is removed. A bony consolidation phase of 6 to 8 weeks ensues, followed by removal of the internal device. The patient is longitudinally followed to track mandibular growth (**Fig. 8**).

Success rate of MDO for relieving airway obstruction is 94%.[38] A systematic review conducted by Master and colleagues[39] compiled complication rates from MDO, including relapse 64.8%, tooth injury 22.5%, hypertrophic scarring 15.6%, nerve injury 11.4%, infection 9.5%, inappropriate distraction vector 8.8%, device failure 7.9%, fusion error 2.4%, and temporomandibular joint injury 0.7%. Predictors of failure include preoperative intubation, gastroesophageal reflux, low birth weight, syndromic diagnosis, neurologic anomalies, intact palate, airway anomalies other than laryngomalacia, and late surgery.[38] Transition to oral feeding occurs in 82% of distracted patients within 12 months postoperatively; however,

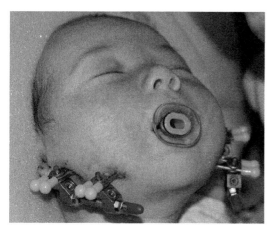

Fig. 6. External distraction allows for multivector changes to the mandible, although having multiple pieces of exposed hardware poses a chronic infectious burden.

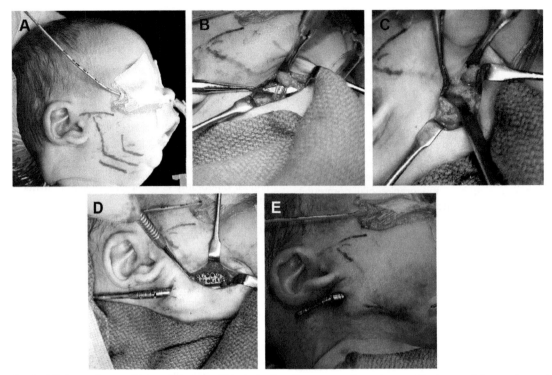

Fig. 7. (*A*) Operative markings of the mandible including the zygomatic arch, mandibular condyle, angle, and proposed submandibular incision, which should be placed at least 1 cm caudal to the inferior mandibular border to avoid injury to the marginal mandibular facial nerve branch. (*B*) Facial artery and vein may be encountered during the soft tissue dissection and exposure of the mandible. (*C*) Completion of the bicortical mandibular osteotomies with mobilization of the distal and mesial segments. (*D*) Application of a uni-vector, semi-buried mandibular distractor to the osteotomized mandible. (*E*) Soft tissue closure of the submandibular incision and application of a universal joint to the extruded distractor arm.

syndromic patients are 5 times more likely to require adjunctive feeding.[40]

TREATMENT PROTOCOL

Universal agreement with respect to diagnosis and management of PRS has yet to be achieved. Lack of randomized controlled trials, limited patient population, training disparities, suboptimal standardization of published studies, and individual biases impede standardization of care.

Evaluation of the patient with PRS begins with history and physical examination by otolaryngology, pulmonology, neonatology, genetics, and plastic surgery. Patients are monitored in a neonatal intensive care unit with continuous pulse oximetry recording desaturation episodes, followed by a formal sleep study to stratify the degree of obstruction. Consideration is placed toward feeding status, weight gain, and desaturation episodes with feeding. Feeding difficulty in the absence of desaturation is addressed by nasogastric feeds and swallow studies.

Desaturation on clinical examination and abnormal polysomnography prompt a comprehensive airway examination with nasoendoscopy and bronchoscopy to evaluate for synchronous lesions. Those with subglottic obstruction may have a suboptimal response to TLA or MDO and undergo tracheostomy.

Tongue-base obstruction is managed with increasing invasiveness. Nonsurgical maneuvers, such as prone and lateral positioning, nasopharyngeal stenting, and noninvasive CPAP, are trialed. Should this fail, the senior author performs MDO in accordance with certain centers[41,42]; however, others may elect to pursue TLA initially, reserving MDO only for those who have failed TLA.[43]

In a recent survey of surgeon members of the American Cleft Palate-Craniofacial Association, nearly half preferred MDO as first-line treatment for airway obstruction.[44] Some advocate for a predictive management algorithm as a function of the maxillo-mandibular discrepancy, severity of glossoptosis, persistent desaturations with prone positioning, feeding difficulties, nasogastric tube dependence, concomitant airway anomalies, and failure of nonsurgical management.[44]

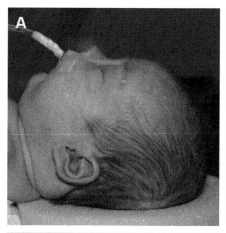

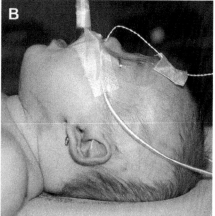

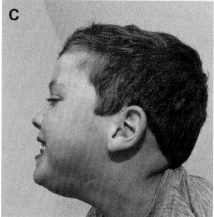

Fig. 8. Lateral view of patient. (*A*) Before mandibular distraction, demonstrating the markedly retrognathic mandible. (*B*) After consolidation, with slight prognathism and well-healed submandibular incision. (*C*) Following years of healing and further mandibular growth with sustained maxillo-mandibular relationship.

Although some centers argue for stratification of severity of obstruction as a node in the decision tree between pursuing TLA versus MDO, others consistently perform TLA as a first-line treatment, reserving MDO for failure of TLA.[43,44] As referenced earlier, a growing majority of craniofacial surgeons view MDO as definitive treatment of airway obstruction, excluding TLA from their management algorithm.[41,42] In light of the variability in diagnostic criteria and disagreement concerning the role of MDO and TLA in the surgical management of PRS, further multicenter work should be undertaken toward achieving a standardized treatment protocol.

SUMMARY

PRS is the clinical triad of micrognathia, glossoptosis, and airway obstruction found within a diverse spectrum of nonsyndromic and syndromic patients. A comprehensive evaluation by a multidisciplinary team helps to establish a diagnosis and guide treatment. Nonsurgical positional and nasopharyngeal stenting maneuvers should be trialed before surgical intervention. Airway interventions must be undertaken only after nasoendoscopy and bronchoscopy to delineate sites of airway compromise beyond the tongue base, as patients with subglottic anomalies may be poor candidates for distraction and should undergo tracheostomy. Surgical options include TLA, subperiosteal FMR, and MDO. Disagreement remains invariant among institutions regarding a uniform treatment algorithm for this diverse group of patients.

SUPPLEMENTARY DATA

Supplementary data related to this article can be found online at https://doi.org/10.1016/j.cps. 2018.11.010.

REFERENCES

1. Von Siebold E. Micrognathia with breathing problems. Siebold's J (Göttingen) 1835;XV:18.
2. Robin P. La glossoptose. Son diagnostic, ses conséquences, son traitement. Bull Acad Natl Med 1923; 89:37–41.

3. Bütow K-W, Zwahlen RA, Morkel JA, et al. Pierre Robin sequence: subdivision, data, theories, and treatment - Part 1: history, subdivisions, and data. Ann Maxillofac Surg 2016;6(1): 31–4.

4. Vatlach S, Maas C, Poets CF. Birth prevalence and initial treatment of Robin sequence in Germany: a prospective epidemiologic study. Orphanet J Rare Dis 2014;9:9.

5. Printzlau A, Anderson M. Pierre Robin sequence in Denmark: a retrospective population-based epidemiological study. Cleft Palate Craniofac J 2004; 41(1):47–52.

6. Evans KN, Sie KC, Hopper RA, et al. Robin sequence: from diagnosis to development of an effective management plan. Pediatrics 2011; 127(5):936–48.

7. Bush PG, Williams AJ. Incidence of the Robin anomalad (Pierre Robin syndrome). Br J Plast Surg 1983; 36(4):434–7.

8. Tan TY, Kilpatrick NK, Farlie PG. Developmental and genetic perspectives on Pierre Robin sequence. Am J Med Genet C Semin Med Genet 2013;163C(4): 295–305.

9. Rintala A, Ranta R, Stegars T. On the pathogenesis of cleft palate in the Pierre Robin syndrome. Scand J Plast Reconstr Surg 1984;18(2):237–40.

10. Gomez-Ospina N, Bernstein JA. Clinical, cytogenetic, and molecular outcomes in a series of 66 patients with Pierre Robin sequence and literature review: 22q11.2 deletion is less common than other chromosomal anomalies. Am J Med Genet A 2016; 170A(4):870–80.

11. Jakobsen LP, Ullmann R, Christensen SB, et al. Pierre Robin sequence may be caused by dysregulation of SOX9 and KCNJ2. J Med Genet 2007;44(6): 381–6.

12. Cohen SM, Greathouse ST, Rabbani CC, et al. Robin sequence: what the multidisciplinary approach can do. J Multidiscip Healthc 2017;10:121–32.

13. Kaufman MG, Cassady CI, Hyman CH, et al. Prenatal identification of Pierre Robin sequence: a review of the literature and look towards the future. Fetal Diagn Ther 2016;39(2):81–9.

14. Paladini D, Morra T, Teodoro A, et al. Objective diagnosis of micrognathia in the fetus: the jaw index. Obstet Gynecol 1999;93:382–6.

15. Rogers-Vizena CR, Mulliken JB, Daniels KM. Prenatal features predictive of Robin sequence identified by fetal magnetic resonance imaging. Plast Reconstr Surg 2016;137(6):999e–1006e.

16. Greathouse ST, Costa M, Ferrera A, et al. The surgical treatment of Robin sequence. Ann Plast Surg 2016;77(4):413–9.

17. Sher AE. Mechanisms of airway obstruction in Robin sequence: implications for treatment. Cleft Palate Craniofac J 1992;29(3):224–31.

18. Khansa I, Hall C, Madhoun LL, et al. Airway and feeding outcomes of mandibular distraction, tongue-lip adhesion, and conservative management in Pierre Robin sequence: a prospective study. Plast Reconstr Surg 2017;139(4):975e–83e.

19. Susarla SM, Mundinger GS, Chang CC. Gastrostomy placement rates in infants with Pierre Robin sequence: a comparison of tongue-lip adhesion and mandibular distraction osteogenesis. Plast Reconstr Surg 2017;139(1):149–54.

20. Gangopadhyay N, Mendonca DA, Woo AS. Pierre Robin sequence. Semin Plast Surg 2012;26(2): 76–82.

21. Collins B, Powitzky R, Robledo C. Airway management in Pierre Robin sequence: patterns of practice. Cleft Palate Craniofac J 2014;51(3):283–9.

22. Mackay DR. Controversies in the diagnosis and management of the Robin sequence. J Craniofac Surg 2011;22(2):415–20.

23. Chang AB, Masters IB, Williams GR, et al. A modified nasopharyngeal tube to relieve high upper airway obstruction. Pediatr Pulmonol 2000;29(4): 299–306.

24. Albino FP, Wood BC, Han KD, et al. Clinical factors associated with the non-operative airway management of patients with Robin sequence. Arch Plast Surg 2016;43(6):506–11.

25. Amaddeo A, Abadie V, Chalouhi C, et al. Continuous positive airway pressure for upper airway obstruction in infants with Pierre Robin sequence. Plast Reconstr Surg 2016;137(2):609–12.

26. Huang F, Lo LJ, Chen YR, et al. Tongue-lip adhesion in the management of Pierre Robin sequence with airway obstruction: technique and outcome. Chang Gung Med J 2005;28(2):90–6.

27. Kumar KS, Vylopilli S, Sivadasan A, et al. Tongue-lip adhesion in Pierre Robin sequence. J Korean Assoc Oral Maxillofac Surg 2016;42(1):47–50.

28. Qaqish C, Caccamese FJ. The tongue-lip adhesion. Operat Tech Otolaryngol Head Neck Surg 2009; 20(4):274–7.

29. Viezel-Mathieu A, Safran T, Gilardino MS. A systematic review of the effectiveness of tongue lip adhesion in improving airway obstruction in children with Pierre Robin sequence. J Craniofac Surg 2016;27(6): 1453–6.

30. Kirschner RE, Low DW, Randall P, et al. Surgical airway management in Pierre Robin sequence: is there a role for tongue-lip adhesion? Cleft Palate Craniofac J 2003;40(1):13–8.

31. Camacho M, Noller MW, Zaghi S. Tongue-lip adhesion and tongue repositioning for obstructive sleep apnoea in Pierre Robin sequence: a systematic review and meta-analysis. J Laryngol Otol 2017; 131(5):378–83.

32. Denny AD, Amm CA, Schaefer RB. Outcomes of tongue-lip adhesion for neonatal respiratory distress

caused by Pierre Robin sequence. J Craniofac Surg 2004;15(5):819–23.

33. Delorme RP, Larocque Y, Caouette-Laberge L. Innovative surgical approach for the Pierre Robin anomalad: subperiosteal release of the floor of the mouth musculature. Plast Reconstr Surg 1989; 83(6):960–4.

34. Caouette-Laberge L, Borsuk DE, Bortoluzzi PA. Subperiosteal release of the floor of the mouth to correct airway obstruction in pierre robin sequence: review of 31 cases. Cleft Palate Craniofac J 2012;49(1): 14–20.

35. McCarthy JG, Schreiber J, Karp N. Lengthening the human mandible by gradual distraction. Plast Reconstr Surg 1992;89(1):1–8 [discussion: 9–10].

36. Rachmiel A, Nseir S, Emodi O. External versus internal distraction devices in treatment of obstructive sleep apnea in craniofacial anomalies. Plast Reconstr Surg Glob Open 2014;2(7):e188.

37. Resnick CM. Precise osteotomies for mandibular distraction in infants with Robin sequence using virtual surgical planning. Int J Oral Maxillofac Surg 2018;47(1):35–43.

38. Almajed A, Viezel-Mathieu A, Gilardino MS. Outcome following surgical interventions for micrognathia in infants with Pierre Robin sequence: a systematic review of the literature. Cleft Palate Craniofac J 2017;54(1):32–42.

39. Master DL, Hanson PR, Gosain AK. Complications of mandibular distraction osteogenesis. J Craniofac Surg 2010;21(5):1565–70.

40. Breik O, Umapathysivam K, Tivey D. Feeding and reflux in children after mandibular distraction osteogenesis for micrognathia: a systematic review. Int J Pediatr Otorhinolaryngol 2016;85: 128–35.

41. Ching JA, Daggett JD, Alvarez SA. A simple mandibular distraction protocol to avoid tracheostomy in patients with Pierre Robin sequence. Cleft Palate Craniofac J 2017;54(2):210–5.

42. Paes EC, van Nunen D, Speleman L, et al. A pragmatic approach to infants with Robin sequence: a retrospective cohort study and presence of a treatment algorithm. Clin Oral Investig 2015;19(8):2101–14.

43. Schaefer RB, Stadler JA, Gosain AK. To distract or not to distract: an algorithm for airway management in isolated Pierre Robin sequence. Plast Reconstr Surg 2004;113(4):1113–25.

44. Wai-Yee L, Poon A, Courtemanche D, et al. Airway management in Pierre Robin sequence: the Vancouver classification. Plast Surg (Oakv) 2017;25(1): 14–20.

Pediatric Craniomaxillofacial Oncologic Reconstruction

Robert F. Dempsey, MD[a], Daniel C. Chelius Jr, MD[b],
William C. Pederson, MD[a], Marco Maricevich, MD[a],
Amy L. Dimachkieh, MD[b], Michael E. Kupferman, MD[c],
Howard L. Weiner, MD[d], Larry H. Hollier Jr, MD[a],
Edward P. Buchanan, MD[a],*

KEYWORDS

- Pediatric reconstruction • Pediatric oncology • Pediatric head and face tumors
- Virtual surgical planning • Pediatric microsurgery • Pediatric craniofacial surgery

KEY POINTS

- Pediatric craniomaxillofacial oncologic reconstruction creates unique challenges compared with adults.
- Future growth, limited available donor sites and associated morbidity, and the increased technical challenges of smaller donor tissues must be considered in pediatric reconstruction.
- Early and open communication between ablative and reconstructive surgeons is critical to success.
- Virtual surgical planning is helpful in modeling anticipated defects and subsequent reconstruction with customized implants.
- Dental restoration should be deferred until skeletal maturity to accommodate the adult dental arch.

INTRODUCTION

Fortunately, compared with their adult counterparts, the incidence of malignant and benign neoplasms of the head and face requiring radical resection in the pediatric population is low. However, when these cases are encountered they create unique challenges to reconstruction. This is caused by several factors including the need to account for future growth, limited available donor sites and associated morbidity, and the increased technical challenges of smaller donor tissues.

In general, the head and face are divided into vertical thirds. The superior third consists of the forehead, scalp, and calvarium. The middle third consists of the midface including the orbit, zygoma, palate, and maxilla. The lower third consists primarily of the mandible. Much has been written about reconstruction algorithms in the adult population to address these areas.[1–6] Although these are useful guides when considering reconstruction in the pediatric patient, they are not directly applicable for the reasons listed previously. We have experienced a recent increase in pediatric

Disclosure Statement: The authors have nothing to disclose.
[a] Division of Plastic Surgery, Michael E. DeBakey Department of Surgery, Baylor College of Medicine, 6701 Fannin Street, CC 610.00, Houston, TX 77030, USA; [b] Pediatric Otolaryngology–Head and Neck Surgery, Baylor College of Medicine, 6701 Fannin Street, Suite 540, Houston, TX 77030, USA; [c] Department of Head and Neck Surgery, Division of Surgery, The University of Texas MD Anderson Cancer Center, 1515 Holcombe Boulevard, Ste 1445, Houston, TX 77030, USA; [d] Division of Pediatric Neurosurgery, Michael E. DeBakey Department of Surgery, Baylor College of Medicine, 6701 Fannin Street, Suite 1230.01, Houston, TX 77030, USA
* Corresponding author.
E-mail address: ebuchana@bcm.edu

Clin Plastic Surg 46 (2019) 261–273
https://doi.org/10.1016/j.cps.2018.11.011
0094-1298/19/© 2018 Elsevier Inc. All rights reserved.

patients at our center requiring craniomaxillofacial reconstruction following tumor extirpation and present our experience and treatment considerations with representative case examples next.

PREOPERATIVE CONSIDERATIONS

As with any other multidisciplinary surgery, open communication between services is critical when creating the preoperative reconstructive plan. Doing so ensures a well-coordinated case with all steps clearly delineated and agreed on beforehand by the team members. This includes the proper sequence of tumor extirpation and specimen handoff. Equally important is open communication with the patient and family to set realistic expectations of postoperative outcomes, potential complications, need for short-term tracheostomy versus long-term intubation, anticipated perioperative hospital stay, and often the need for staged procedures.

Knowledge of the anticipated defect size, missing tissue types, need for bony reconstruction, adequacy of intraoperative margin analysis, and anticipated adjuvant therapies all need to be considered preoperatively. Most frequently, free flap harvest can occur simultaneously with tumor extirpation. However, it is important to have separate setups and nursing or surgical technologist assistants to avoid iatrogenic seeding of tumor cells in the donor site.

Finally, adequate time is required before surgery to appropriately plan a complex reconstruction. Virtual surgical planning (VSP) has proved an invaluable tool to better understand the anticipated defect when creating a reconstructive plan. Often, models are used in this regard, and custom plates and implants to promote increased intraoperative efficiency. Although industry turnover for these devices continues to improve, currently 1 to 2 weeks is required before these tools are available for surgery. Thus, once the need for complex reconstruction is identified by the ablative surgeon, the patient should be promptly referred to and evaluated by the reconstructive surgeon.

UPPER THIRD

Depending on level of invasion, extirpation of a tumor in the upper third of the head may leave a defect in the scalp, calvarium, or both. Reconstruction of soft tissue only defects follow a similar algorithm to those seen in adult patients based on the size of the defect. Care should be taken to delay reconstruction until adequate negative margins are confirmed on final pathology. Primary closure is often possible for defects up to 3 cm (in children older than 5–6 year old) with wide subgaleal undermining, avoiding the need for any donor site morbidity. Larger defects require additional tissue in the form of skin grafts, local pedicled flaps, or free flaps.

Split thickness skin grafts (STSG) may be used to reconstruct either the primary defect or donor site of a local flap. They require a well vascularized bed, usually pericranium. Although grafts are usually placed without meshing for cosmesis, alopecia and color mismatch are expected sequelae. However, these may be later addressed with secondary reconstruction using tissue-expanded hair-bearing scalp flaps.

In the absence of an adequate vascularized bed, dermal regenerative templates may be considered and applied directly over denuded bone. These offer several advantages of allowing subsequent skin graft reconstruction over a previously nonvascularized surface, use of a thinner split thickness autograft, and improving contour irregularity between the native and reconstructed scalp. However, these products greatly increase the cost of reconstruction, require a period of 2 to 3 weeks of negative pressure dressings to promote vascular ingrowth, and consequently should be considered on a case-by-case basis.

Local flaps may be raised on any number of axial blood supplies of the richly vascularized scalp. Furthermore, they may be raised as either full or partial thickness. Partial thickness flaps do not disturb the skin or hair of the donor site and include pericranial or galeal flaps, which may be used to resurface a previously nonvascularized wound bed for immediate STSG. Full thickness flaps carry hair-bearing skin and are usually raised in a subgaleal plane to allow STSG over the donor site pericranium if they are unable to be closed primarily. Long, wide flaps are required to provide adequate coverage of the defect, which is easily underestimated, and facilitate rotation. Larger defects may call for bipedicled "bucket handled" flaps to provide adequate coverage, but offer less mobility.

Extremely large defects (>9 cm) without vascularized graftable wound beds are usually unamenable to local flap coverage and require free tissue transfer. These may be fasciocutaneous, myocutaneous, or muscle-only free flaps.

Because harvesting a skin paddle of this size usually precludes primary closure of the donor site, muscle-only flaps with STSG are favored to minimize donor site dyscosmesis. Flap selection is dictated by defect size and required pedicle length for vascular anastomosis. The superficial temporal vessels are favored as recipient vessels because of their proximity of the defect. However, they may not be available if included in the excision specimen, of inadequate size in a young child, or occasionally absent. In these scenarios dissection is carried into the neck to make use of the facial vessels. This requires a significantly longer pedicle and/or interposition vein grafts. Because of this potential variability, the latissimus dorsi and rectus abdominis have become the workhorse muscle flaps for reconstruction of large scalp defects. Although they present significant bulk at time of inset, they demonstrate appreciable atrophy over time.

Calvarial reconstruction presents another set of challenges. In general, autologous cranioplasty is always favorable to alloplastic reconstruction in that it offers excellent osseointegration and growth potential. The most common donor site for autologous cranioplasty is the unaffected skull in the form of full or split thickness grafts and particulate bone grafts. These offer multiple advantages including ready availability in the same field as the defect and lower rates of resorption than bone grafts harvested from other locations.[7]

Full thickness grafts offer excellent coverage of the defect. However, donor site morbidity may be unacceptably high for large defects and rigid calvarial bone grafts are difficult to contour. This may be mitigated by splitting the graft and using half to reconstruct the donor site. The graft may be split ex vivo or in situ; however, the later possess significant technical challenges. Traditionally, the outer table is used for reconstruction of the defect, and inner table for the donor site. However, pediatric calvarium is frequently too thin to split because of absent diploic space, which does not form until 3 to 5 years of age.

For large defects in children with thin donor skull, reconstruction is then performed via exchange cranioplasty. This entails harvest of a full thickness graft to reconstruct the defect and particulate bone from the inner table of the graft to reconstruct the donor site. The particulate bone is frequently secured with an overlying absorbable plate. This has proven highly effective in this age group because of

the high osteogenic potential of the developing skull.[8,9]

Case 1

A 22-month-old boy was referred to our team for evaluation of a left-sided temporoparietal scalp mass, which had been recently enlarging. Biopsy demonstrated a desmoid tumor for which radical resection was recommended by the neurosurgical and otolaryngology teams and subsequent reconstruction by plastic surgery. Based on preoperative imaging, a full thickness defect including scalp and skull with dural preservation measuring 12 cm was anticipated.

The mass was successfully excised en bloc including a large portion of underlying skull. No dural invasion was appreciated. The resultant defect measured 11 cm in maximum dimension. Negative bony margins were unable to be confirmed intraoperatively, so a temporary negative pressure dressing was applied over a resorbable plate (**Fig. 1**).

After confirmation of negative bony margins on permanent pathology, the patient underwent definitive reconstruction via exchange cranioplasty using inner table particulate graft to reconstruct the contralateral parietal donor site and scalp reconstruction with an ipsilateral latissimus dorsi and serratus anterior chimeric muscle free flap anastomosed end-to-end to the superficial temporal artery and vein and STSG. The patient required an unexpected return to the operating room for flap venous thrombosis on postoperative Day 5, which was successfully salvaged with excision of the thrombosed segment and interposition reverse saphenous vein graft. We believe this was likely caused by poor patient compliance with positioning while weaning sedation. No additional complications were encountered. The reconstruction was well healed at 5 months follow-up. Further scalp reconstruction for alopecia with tissue expanders is currently planned (**Fig. 2**).

MIDDLE THIRD

Reconstruction of the middle third of the face in the pediatric patient is often the most challenging because of the need to account for future maxillofacial growth, permanent dentition, facial symmetry, and donor site morbidity.[10] Soft tissue–only defects after resection are often effectively managed through either local tissue or free tissue options. However, the aggressive nature of many pediatric facial tumors often

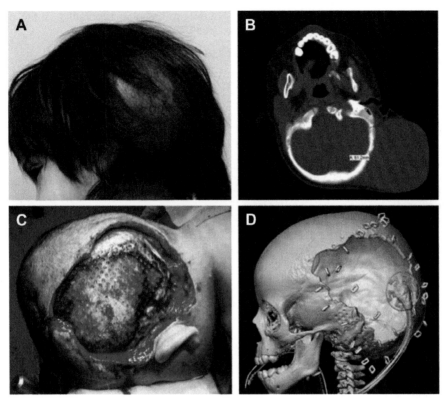

Fig. 1. Case 1: upper third preoperative reconstruction. (*A*) Enlarging left temporoparietal desmoid tumor in a 22-month-old boy. (*B*) Local invasion into the underlying skull is demonstrated on preoperative axial computed tomography (CT) scan. (*C*) Appearance of defect before definitive reconstruction following a period of negative pressure dressing therapy until negative bony margins were confirmed. A resorbable plate was used for neural protection. (*D*) Three-dimensional (3D) reconstruction of postoperative CT scan following tumor resection demonstrating bony defect before definitive reconstruction.

requires maxillary resection because of either direct invasion or to obtain adequate negative margins. Successful reconstruction of these complicated defects of the midface requires consideration of specific reconstructive goals: wound closure, restoration of the barrier between the sinonasal cavity and anterior cranial fossa, separation of the oral and orbital cavities from the sinonasal cavity, support of the orbital contents with maintenance of globe position, oral continence, speech, mastication, avoidance of extropion, maintenance of a patent nasal airway, and restoration of facial harmony.[2]

Defects involving only the soft tissues of the midface are generally found intraorally, and specifically in the palate. Thus, palatoplasty techniques are highly effective to achieve wound closure and maintenance of speech. Even if the hard palate is involved in the resection specimen, soft tissue separation of the oral and sinonasal cavities is often sufficient without boney reconstruction. Defects that cannot be closed with

palatoplasty techniques alone are often amenable to local flap reconstruction via buccal myomucosal flaps. Extremely large defects occasionally require free tissue transfer with common donor sites including the radial forearm, anterolateral thigh, and latissimus dorsi with associated skin paddles.

Classification and reconstruction of limited to full maxillectomy defects in the adult population have been previously well classified.[1,2] Although it is generally accepted that reconstruction should be performed at the same time as resection, full reconstruction may not be possible depending on patient age. The maxilla undergoes dramatic anteroposterior and vertical expansion during the first 5 to 6 years of life, with an almost equal amount of expansion in the ensuing 12 years until facial maturity (**Fig. 3**).[11] Maxillary growth is also associated with growth of the mandible and basal skull, thus maxillary resection in the growing patient can lead to impaired development of all three structures.[12] To minimize these

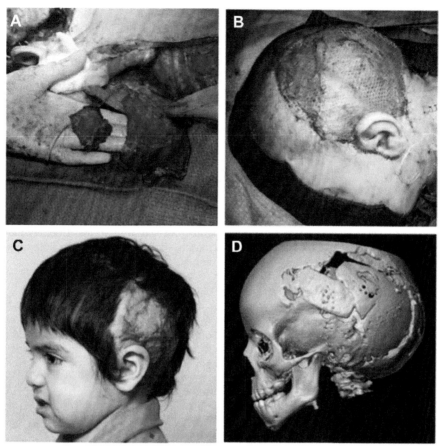

Fig. 2. Case 1: upper third intraoperative and postoperative reconstruction. (*A*) Harvest of an ipsilateral latissimus dorsi and serratus anterior chimeric muscle free flap for scalp reconstruction. (*B*) Free flap inset with split thickness skin graft over exchange cranioplasty. (*C*) Five-month postoperative result with expected alopecia at reconstruction site. (*D*) Five-month postoperative 3D CT of exchange cranioplasty reconstruction.

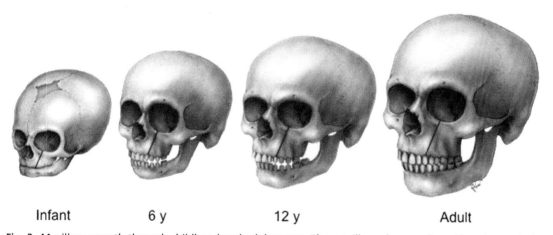

Infant   6 y   12 y   Adult

Fig. 3. Maxillary growth through childhood and adolescence. The maxilla undergoes dramatic anteroposterior and vertical expansion during the first 5 to 6 years of life, with an almost equal amount of expansion in the ensuing 12 years until facial maturity. Note the vertical maxillary height (indicated by the *red line*) nearly doubles between infancy and the age of 6, and then doubles again at facial skeletal maturity. Image created by Katherine Relyea, MS, CMI and printed with permission from Baylor College of Medicine.

adverse consequences, restoration of maxillary-mandibular occlusion is prioritized. However, because permanent dental restoration is usually deferred until skeletal maturity due to unpredictable future facial growth, serial orthodontic prostheses may be used to prevent major asymmetry.

Free flaps have become the gold standard for adult maxillofacial defects and subsequently been successfully applied to pediatric reconstruction with the first reported application in the 1970s using free groin flaps.[10,13–15] Since then, especially for composite defects, free flap donor sites now primarily arise from the fibula, iliac crest, and scapula. The free fibula and iliac crest flaps are particularly well suited for eventual dental implants.

When present, reconstruction of orbital floor defects is dictated by size. Autologous bone is always preferable and bone grafts are usually sufficient.[2] However, extremely large defects and those also involving the zygoma may require reinforcement with alloplastic implants. The most common donor site for these bone grafts is from the parietal skull, which may be taken as either a full thickness, split cortical, or particulate shave graft. The ultimate goal of any orbital reconstruction is to support the globe in a natural position to avoid subsequent diplopia. Alternatively, if exenteration is necessary, the focus becomes creation of an accommodating socket for eventual prosthesis.

Currently, we advocate a two-staged approach to total maxillary defects involving the orbit, zygoma, and palate. The first stage focuses on free flap reconstruction of the orbital floor and zygoma in addition to separating the oral and nasal cavities. We then defer second stage reconstruction closer to skeletal maturity with an osseous-only free fibula flap to match the dental arch for subsequent dental implants.

Case 2

A 14-year-old boy presented with an enlarging 2-cm right hemipalatal mass. Biopsy demonstrated a mucoepidermoid carcinoma, which did not seem to invade the hard palate on preoperative

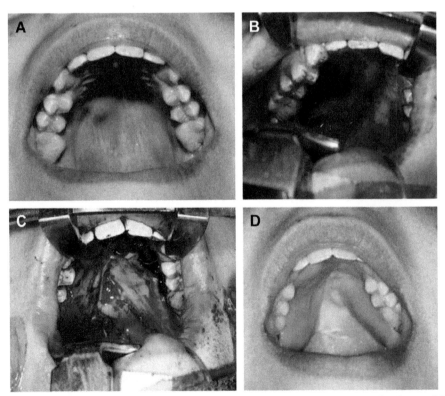

Fig. 4. Case 2: middle third palatal reconstruction. (*A*) Preoperative view of right hemipalatal mass. (*B*) Resulting 2.5-cm defect after tumor extirpation. (*C*) Immediate result after reconstruction with bilateral buccal myomucosal flaps. (*D*) One-year follow-up showing complete healing of reconstruction before pedicle division.

imaging. No evidence of metastasis was detected during staging, thus wide local excision was believed possible. Intraoperatively, the mass was found just crossing midline with hard palatal remodeling without bony invasion. All margins, including nerve margins in palatine fossa, were found to be negative on frozen section. The resultant defect measured 2.5 cm with intact nasal lining and was reconstructed with bilateral buccal myomucosal flaps based at the level of the retromolar trigone and extending anteriorly to oral commissure. He had an uncomplicated postoperative recovery, discharged on postoperative Day 3 after demonstrating adequate oral intake, and remains cancer free on surveillance. Although not interfering with occlusion, he requested pedicle division for comfort, which was performed uneventfully 14 months after reconstruction (**Fig. 4**).

Case 3

An 8-year-old boy was referred to our team for evaluation of a recurrent right orbital meduloepithelioma, which had been previously resected via subtotal exenteration at an outside facility. Completion orbital exenteration was recommended to include the orbital apex and lamina papyracae. Tumor extirpation resulted in a denuded orbit in need of soft tissue reconstruction to resurface the socket for eventual prosthesis. This was accomplished with a contralateral radial forearm free flap, harvested during extirpation, anastomosed to the superior thyroid artery and facial vein. The donor site was reconstructed in a staged fashion with Integra and subsequent thin STSG to minimize the defect. He had no postoperative complications and currently is awaiting prosthesis fitting (**Fig. 5**).

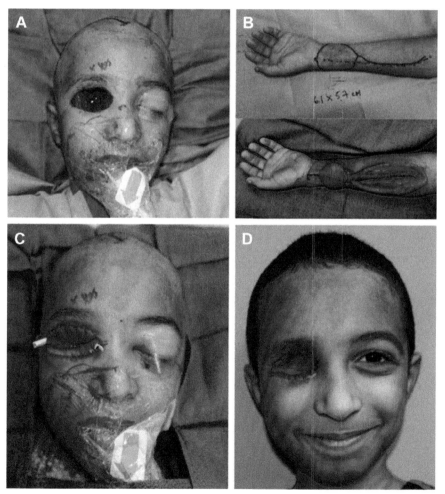

Fig. 5. Case 3: middle third orbital reconstruction. (*A*) Right orbital defect after extirpation extending to orbital apex. (*B*) Left radial forearm free flap design and harvest. (*C*) Immediate on-table result after flap inset. (*D*) Two-month follow-up awaiting fitting for prosthesis on return in 6 months.

Case 4

A 15-year-old girl was referred to our team for evaluation of a rapidly enlarging left maxillary mass, initially misdiagnosed as an odontogenic abscess. Subsequent biopsy demonstrated an extraskeletal mesenchymal chondrosarcoma. After favorable response to neoadjuvant chemotherapy, extirpation was planned with the aid of VSP. The anticipated left hemimaxillectomy defect included the left orbital floor and zygoma, thus reconstruction with a Polyether Ether Ketone (PEEK) was designed (**Fig. 6**). Soft tissue reconstruction to separate the oral, nasal, and orbital cavities was planned with a free anterolateral thigh flap. Because of the already complicated nature of the reconstruction and anticipated need for adjuvant radiation

therapy, bony reconstruction of the left dental arch was deferred. The patient underwent successful extirpation, reconstruction, and temporary tracheostomy without complications. She was successfully decanulated on postoperative Day 9 and discharged home 4 days later following swallow evaluation and demonstrating adequate oral intake. We plan an osseous-only free fibula free flap reconstruction following adjuvant therapies to accommodate eventual dental implants (**Fig. 7**).

Case 5

A 16-year-old boy was referred for maxillary reconstruction following previous left hemimaxillectomy for fibrous dysplasia at an outside institution at the age of 12. His soft tissue defect was

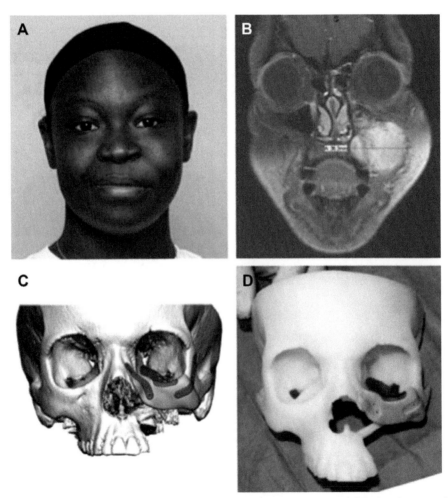

Fig. 6. Case 4: middle third composite first stage preoperative reconstruction. (*A*) Preoperative photograph following neoadjuvant chemotherapy just before surgery demonstrating a left facial mass. (*B*) T1-weighted MRI demonstrating a left maxillary mesenchymal chondrosarcoma. (*C*) VSP of anticipated defect allowing prefabrication of PEEK implant to reconstruct excised left orbital floor and zygoma. (*D*) Fabricated custom PEEK implant on model.

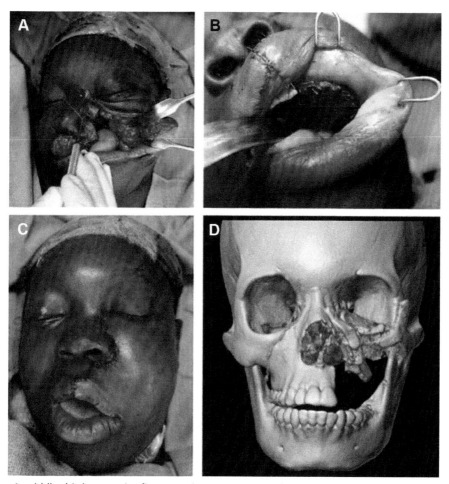

Fig. 7. Case 4: middle third composite first stage intraoperative and postoperative reconstruction. (*A*) Resultant defect following tumor extirpation. (*B*) Inset of anterolateral fasciocutaneous free flap over PEEK orbital floor reconstruction to separate oral, nasal, and orbital cavities. (*C*) Immediate, on-table, result following closure of Weber Ferguson incision. (*D*) Postoperative Day 10 3D CT demonstrating PEEK left orbital floor and zygoma reconstruction.

reconstructed with an ipsilateral latissimus dorsi free flap without complications at the time of extirpation. VSP was used to design an osseous-only fibula free flap to match his adult dental arch and custom plate to inset the flap. Additionally, a hemi–Le Fort I osteotomy was planned to reposition the right maxillary remnant into occlusion with this mandibular dentition using a custom splint because it had collapsed medially. Once healed, the fibula will function to accommodate dental implants to restore his maxillary dentition (**Fig. 8**).

LOWER THIRD

Reconstruction of the lower third of the face centers around the mandible. The mandibular growth center is located in the condylar epiphysis. Because epiphyseal fusion does not occur until 13 to 15 years of age, mandibular resections before fusion results in marked asymmetry if not reconstructed.[16] Therefore, restoration of condylar-basicranial articulation is equally important to maxillary-mandibular occlusion as previously discussed. Again, permanent dental restoration is deferred until skeletal maturity.

Small defects, less than 3 to 5 cm depending on the size of the child, may be reconstructed with nonvascularized bone grafts, which are most frequently harvested from the rib. These usually adequately grow with the patient, although overgrowth has occasionally been reported.[17,18] In extremely young patients (younger than 2 years

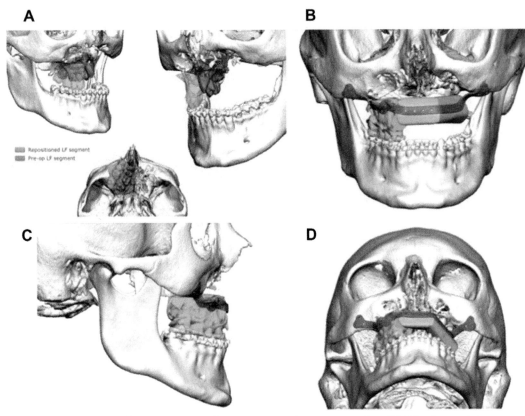

Fig. 8. Case 5: middle third composite second stage preoperative reconstruction. (*A*) VSP of second stage osseous-only free fibula maxillary reconstruction. To obtain normal occlusion, the right maxillary remnant requires repositioning because it had collapsed without dental arch support. The current right maxillary position is shown in *red* and the planned repositioned segment in *blue*. (*B*) Anteroposterior view of the repositioned maxillary remnant (*blue*) with osseous-only fibula free flap (*green*) inset with a custom plate to reconstruct the left maxillary dental arch for eventual implants. (*C*) Right lateral view demonstrating Angle class one occlusion of the repositioned right hemi–Le Fort I segment. (*D*) Worm's eye view of the reconstruction.

of age) with inadequate donor sites, a staged approach using a temporary reconstruction plate with subsequent reconstruction via sagittal split osteotomy or distraction osteogenesis may be required.[10,19]

Larger defects require vascularized bone, which is primarily obtained from the fibula and has become the gold standard in mandible reconstruction for patients as young as 2 years of age. Reliable mandible reconstruction in these young patients is greatly facilitated through the use of custom plates, which allow reliable reproduction of the normal anatomy. This is crucial to maximizing postoperative function, especially if the condyle is to be removed in the tumor specimen. The plate is then removed after 1 year, which we have found to allow adequate healing and incorporation of the fibula free flap, while at the same time not restricting future growth. Final reconstruction

with regards to dentition is deferred until skeletal maturity to accommodate adult dentition and allow correction of any interval growth restriction.

Although rib bone grafts have been reported to occasionally overgrow the contralateral side, fibula free flaps have been reported to not grow sufficiently as the child ages.[19,20] Nonetheless, pediatric free fibula mandible reconstruction has several benefits compared with adults including a more compliant soft tissue envelope with better flap adaptation because of the increased neural plasticity.[10,20]

Case 6

A 2-year-old girl presented with an enlarging left mandibular mass. Subsequent biopsy was unable to delineate between a benign desmoid fibromatosis versus malignant fibrosarcoma. Thus, left hemimandibulectomy with sentinel lymph node biopsy was recommended. Temporary tracheostomy was also discussed with the family to ensure a secure perioperative airway. Left condylar resection was deemed unlikely based on preoperative imaging. VSP was used to model the anticipated defect, create cutting guides for the required 13-cm osseous-only fibula free flap, and a custom plate for flap inset. The flap was harvested from the ipsilateral leg during tumor extirpation and sentinel lymph node biopsy. The flap was then secured to the custom plate, inset to the residual right hemimandible and left subcondylar remnant, and anastomosed to the facial vessels (**Fig. 9**).

The patient had an uneventful hospital course, spending 7 days in the intensive care unit (slightly longer than average because of fresh tracheostomy protocol). She was successfully decanulated on postoperative Day 15 and discharged the following day tolerating adequate oral intake after swallow evaluation. The titanium plate was removed uneventfully 10 months later with demonstration of complete healing and osseous integration of the fibula free flap into the mandibular remnants. Final pathology demonstrated

desmoid fibromatosis and she has remained without evidence of recurrent disease and good masticatory function after 2 years of follow-up (**Fig. 10**).

POSTOPERATIVE CONSIDERATIONS

Postoperative care is as important to a successful outcome as preoperative planning and intraoperative execution. Flap loss is rare, but usually related to either the technical challenges of anastomosing comparatively smaller pediatric vessels or poor compliance with postoperative immobilization.[13] For this reason, we keep our patients sedated during the critical first 72 hours of re-endothelialization. Sedation is then slowly weaned while maintaining adequate analgesia after ensuring flap viability. The patient is subsequently extubated/decanulated when deemed medically appropriate by the critical care and otolaryngology teams. Overall, our patients typically spend 4 to 5 days in the intensive care unit and an approximately equal amount of time in a nonmonitored setting. They are discharged home after demonstrating adequate swallow function and adequate oral intake.

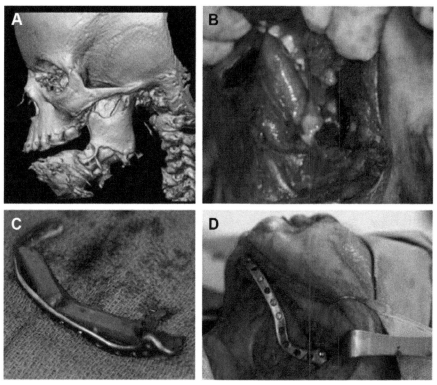

Fig. 9. Case 6: lower third preoperative and intraoperative reconstruction. (*A*) Preoperative 3D CT scan used for VSP to model anticipated defect and custom plate fabrication. (*B*) On table left hemimandibulectomy defect with preserved left subcondylar remnant. (*C*) Left osseous-only fibula free flap secured to custom plate. (*D*) Free flap secured to mandibular remnants and anastomosed to readily available facial vessels.

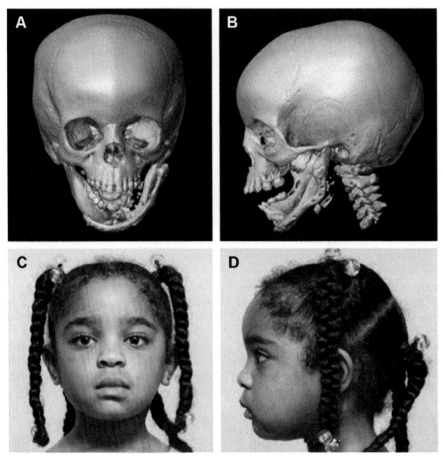

Fig. 10. Case 6: lower third postoperative reconstruction. (*A*) Anteroposterior view of 10-month postoperative 3D CT scan demonstrating osseous union before hardware removal. (*B*) Left lateral view of postoperative 3D CT scan. (*C*) Two-year result after hardware removal demonstrating lower facial symmetry, and (*D*) preserved jaw line.

SUMMARY

Reconstruction of defects of the head and face in the pediatric population requires special consideration for future growth, and at times temporization in anticipation for skeletal maturity followed by subsequent reoperation at an appropriate age. Additional challenges include more limited donor sites, smaller anastomoses, and unpredictable postoperative compliance compared with their adult counterparts. Nonetheless, successful composite bony and soft tissue, and isolated soft tissue defects in children are safely reconstructed using existing local tissue and microsurgical techniques.

REFERENCES

1. Hanasono MM, Silva AK, Yu P, et al. A comprehensive algorithm for oncologic maxillary reconstruction. Plast Reconstr Surg 2013;131(1):47–60.

2. McCarthy CM, Cordeiro PG. Microvascular reconstruction of oncologic defects of the midface. Plast Reconstr Surg 2010;126(6):1947–59.

3. Schultz BD, Sosin M, Nam A, et al. Classification of mandible defects and algorithm for microvascular reconstruction. Plast Reconstr Surg 2015;135(4): 743e–54e.

4. Leedy JE, Janis JE, Rohrich RJ. Reconstruction of acquired scalp defects: an algorithmic approach. Plast Reconstr Surg 2005;116(4):54e–72e.

5. Chang EI, Hanasono MM. State-of-the-art reconstruction of midface and facial deformities. J Surg Oncol 2016;113(8):962–70.

6. Uygur S, Eryilmaz T, Cukurluoglu O, et al. Management of cranial bone defects: a reconstructive algorithm according to defect size. J Craniofac Surg 2013;24(5):1606–9.

7. Rogers GF, Greene AK. Autogenous bone graft: basic science and clinical implications. J Craniofac Surg 2012;23(1):323–7.

8. Lam S, Kuether J, Fong A, et al. Cranioplasty for large-sized calvarial defects in the pediatric population: a review. Craniomaxillofac Trauma Reconstr 2015;8(2):159–70.

9. Rogers GF, Greene AK, Mulliken JB, et al. Exchange cranioplasty using autologous calvarial particulate

bone graft effectively repairs large cranial defects. Plast Reconstr Surg 2011;127(4):1631–42.

10. Valentini V, Califano L, Cassoni A, et al. Maxillomandibular reconstruction in pediatric patients: how to do it? J Craniofac Surg 2018;29(3):761–6.

11. Laowansiri U, Behrents RG, Araujo E, et al. Maxillary growth and maturation during infancy and early childhood. Angle Orthod 2013;83(4):563–71.

12. Thilander B. Basic mechanisms in craniofacial growth. Acta Odontol Scand 1995;53(3):144–51.

13. Arnold DJ, Wax MK, Microvascular Committee of the American Academy of Otolaryngology–Head and Neck Surgery. Pediatric microvascular reconstruction: a report from the Microvascular Committee. Otolaryngol Head Neck Surg 2007;136(5):848–51.

14. Harii K, Ohmori K. Free groin flaps in children. Plast Reconstr Surg 1975;55(5):588–92.

15. Valentini V, Cassoni A, Marianetti TM, et al. Anterolateral thigh flap for the reconstruction of head and neck defects: alternative or replacement of the radial forearm flap? J Craniofac Surg 2008;19(4): 1148–53.

16. Genden EM, Buchbinder D, Chaplin JM, et al. Reconstruction of the pediatric maxilla and mandible. Arch Otolaryngol Head Neck Surg 2000; 126(3):293–300.

17. Goerke D, Sampson DE, Tibesar RJ, et al. Rib reconstruction of the absent mandibular condyle in children. Otolaryngol Head Neck Surg 2013; 149(3):372–6.

18. Perrott DH, Umeda H, Kaban LB. Costochondral graft construction/reconstruction of the ramus/condyle unit: long-term follow-up. Int J Oral Maxillofac Surg 1994;23(6 Pt 1):321–8.

19. Guo L, Ferraro NF, Padwa BL, et al. Vascularized fibular graft for pediatric mandibular reconstruction. Plast Reconstr Surg 2008;121(6):2095–105.

20. Phillips JH, Rechner B, Tompson BD. Mandibular growth following reconstruction using a free fibula graft in the pediatric facial skeleton. Plast Reconstr Surg 2005;116(2):419–24 [discussion: 425–6].

Printed and bound by CPI Group (UK) Ltd, Croydon, CR0 4YY

08/05/2025

01864743-0005